A Cup of Comfort
for Mothers to Be

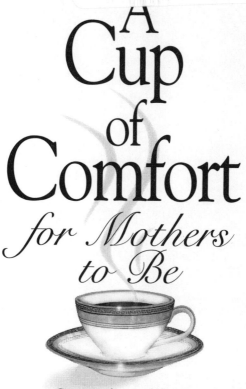

Stories that celebrate
a very special time

EDITED BY
COLLEEN SELL

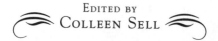

ADAMS MEDIA
Avon, Massachusetts

In loving memory of Blanche Sell, beloved mother of fourteen.

Copyright ©2006 F+W Publications, Inc.
All rights reserved. This book, or parts thereof, may not be
reproduced in any form without permission from the publisher;
exceptions are made for brief excerpts used in published reviews.

A Cup of Comfort is a trademark of F+W Publications, Inc.

Published by
Adams Media, an F+W Publications Company
57 Littlefield Street, Avon, MA 02322. U.S.A.
www.adamsmedia.com and *www.cupofcomfort.com*

ISBN 10: 1-59337-574-3
ISBN 13: 978-1-59337-574-4
Printed in Canada.

J I H G F E D C B A

Library of Congress Cataloging-in-Publication Data
A cup of comfort for mothers to be / edited by Colleen Sell.
    p. cm. -- (A cup of comfort series book)
        ISBN 1-59337-574-3
    1. Motherhood. 2. Pregnancy. 3. Childbirth.
    4. Mothers. I. Sell, Colleen. II. Series.
                HQ759.C97 2006
            306.874'30973--dc22
                2006014713

This publication is designed to provide accurate and authoritative information
with regard to the subject matter covered. It is sold with the understanding that
the publisher is not engaged in rendering legal, accounting, or other professional
advice. If legal advice or other expert assistance is required, the services of a
competent professional person should be sought.

    —From a *Declaration of Principles* jointly adopted by a Committee of the
American Bar Association and a Committee of Publishers and Associations

Many of the designations used by manufacturers and sellers to distinguish
their products are claimed as trademarks. Where those designations appear in
this book and Adams Media was aware of a trademark claim, the designations
have been printed with initial capital letters.

*This book is available at quantity discounts for bulk purchases.
For information, please call 1-800-872-5627.*

Acknowledgments

My deepest gratitude goes to the women whose very personal stories grace these pages, not only for writing great stuff and allowing us to publish it, but also for being such troopers during the long and sometimes arduous process of compiling this book.

A hearty pat on the back goes to Kate Epstein, my chief comrade-in-arms through several volumes of *A Cup of Comfort*, whose steady hand and dry wit I already miss. An appreciative tip of the hat goes to all of the talented, hardworking folks at Adams Media, most notably Kirsten Amann, Laura Daly, Gary Krebs, and Paula Munier.

I most humbly thank all of the *Cup of Comfort* readers for their interest and loyalty.

Contents

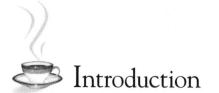 Introduction

"If I had my life to live over, instead of wishing away nine months of pregnancy, I'd have cherished every moment and realized that the wonderment growing inside me was the only chance in life to assist God in a miracle."

—Erma Bombeck

My daughter is newly and unexpectedly pregnant. And I am thrilled. I am also worried. After all, this is my baby giving birth here … my baby, whose own gestation was difficult and whose birth was early and traumatic. My baby girl, who is carrying her second baby while working outside the home full time and while her first baby is still in diapers, still nursing, and still not sleeping through the night. My precious child, who will give birth to Baby #2 when Baby #1—otherwise known as "John," "JB," and "Our Boy"—is but 20 months old. My beloved daughter, whose biochemistry is rather sensitive, and so she endures migraines, nausea, and other unpleasant symptoms during pregnancy, and who did not inherit my child-bearing hips and pelvis, and so is facing another cesarean section. My strong and capable but exhausted and stressed-out daughter, whose husband recently returned to work after an extended and painful and only partial recovery from a serious back injury and several surgeries, leaving these hard-working high-school sweethearts of eighteen years physically, emotionally, and financially spent.

And yet . . . they are, as Susan Townsend, whose story is featured in this book, would say, "partners in a miracle." And they are overjoyed. And cherishing these precious, never-to-be-reclaimed moments. And making it all work, somehow. And so I push aside my worries (most of the time) and instead focus on celebrating this most miraculous and joyous experience with them. I realize that my job, as mother of the mommy and grandma of the grandbabies, is to encourage and support, to help alleviate whatever challenges there may be and accentuate the positive.

Pregnancy, childbirth, and those first few hours and days of being a new mommy to a newborn can be overwhelming and scary—especially if the mother has been bombarded with horror stories and misinformation, or if her fears and concerns have been pooh-poohed, or if things don't go as planned and hoped. I wish for every expectant mother to be surrounded by conscientious mothers and professionals who listen compassionately, advise carefully, and share the wonders of their own pregnancies, childbirths, and new mommy experiences. I wish to be that source of wisdom, hope, and inspiration to my daughter and to other expectant mothers I might encounter. I wish I would have had more of that kind of positive reinforcement during each of my four pregnancies, including the one that resulted in the heartbreak of miscarriage and especially the difficult one that resulted in the miraculous birth of my middle child, now expecting her second child. Still, in looking back, it is the encouraging words of other mothers and the joyful moments I experienced during the pregnancies, births, and homecomings of my three wonderful children that I remember and cherish most.

May the heartwarming stories in this book, written by mothers who have experienced the joys and challenges of pregnancy and childbirth firsthand, bring you comfort and pleasure. And may you be reminded to cherish each miraculous moment of the wonderment growing inside you.

—*Colleen Sell*

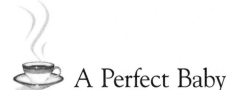# A Perfect Baby

At my six-week postpartum visit, Dr. Wigginton hands me a small box with a pink lid. Inside is a stainless steel, long-handled baby spoon engraved with my daughter's name and birth date.

"Thank you," I say, and then wait, because Dr. Wigginton is looking everywhere except at me, his face pinched with concentration. He is trying, I soon realize, to find the right words; there is something he wants to say.

Finally, he looks at me. "I just . . ." he begins, but it takes two tries. "I just wanted you to have a perfect baby."

Now, I am the one who can't look him in the eye.

Everyone looks forward to the twenty-week ultrasound—to that first glimpse, grainy and shifting, when the ultrasound tech says things you've been waiting so long to hear: "It's a boy," or, "See that, she's sucking her thumb," or, "Oh look, toes!"

I took a videotape to my ultrasound so that my husband could see it later. He'd planned to come, but our older daughter woke up with a fever of 102, so we decided to cancel the sitter, and he stayed home instead.

So, I was there alone to hear, "Looks like a girl," and "There's her heart," and "Wait right there, I want the doctor to see this."

I laid on that table for far too long while the doctor and the ultrasound nurse searched and searched for what they weren't seeing, and examined and re-examined what they were seeing. They couldn't find my baby girl's diaphragm, the muscle that supports the organs in the chest; they couldn't find lung tissue. They did find a small anomaly—Dr. Wigginton called it a cyst—in my baby's brain.

That's just not how twenty-week ultrasounds are supposed to go.

At home, I looked up diaphragmatic hernias—conditions in which the diaphragm doesn't form properly in the developing fetus. What I found was scary; half to three-quarters of such babies die. Mortality is higher for girls (like mine), for babies with multiple problems (that troubling cyst in her brain), and for babies with low birth weights (at one point the doctor had extended my due date three weeks based on her size, but I told them they had to be wrong; she was just small, for some reason).

I also looked up pulmonary agenesis—the condition where one or both lungs fail to form. Bilateral (both sides) pulmonary agenesis is exceedingly rare; there were only eleven recorded cases worldwide as of that year. The sources I read stated that the condition was "generally incompatible with life." Unilateral pulmonary agenesis is very rare, too, but is more common than bilateral and usually accompanied by other developmental defects of varying severity. Either is worse than a diaphragmatic hernia. I feared that I would be case number twelve in recorded history of a woman whose baby was born without lungs; that not only would I have to bury my baby, but that I'd also have to spend the next thirty years fending off scientists wanting to study my case.

Friends and relatives offered what support they could, but it wasn't much. We were on everyone's prayer list. My grandparents offered us one of their burial plots, should we need it. It was the only concrete thing anyone could do.

The latest imaging technique at the time was the three-dimensional ultrasound. I read articles about this technological wonder that could give you a sepia-toned image of your unborn baby's face. In larger cities, women could go to the mall and have their baby's "portrait" imaged for several hundred dollars. In out-of-the-way western Kentucky, the only way I was going to have access to such a wonder was to need it. At twenty-five weeks, my husband and I traveled out of state to the nearest perinatologist's office, where I laid for hours on a table while my baby was poked and prodded, measured and examined, first by a technician, then by the doctor herself—a youthful, smartly dressed woman whose name was Turnquest-Wells.

Dr. Turnquest-Wells said, "What we're seeing is a neural tube defect, a condition called 'spina bifida'—"

Spina bifida? Not pulmonary agenesis? Not diaphragmatic hernia?

I said, "But she has lungs?"

Dr. Turnquest-Wells seemed taken aback. "Um, yes," she said.

"And she has a whole diaphragm?" I asked.

"Uh, well, yes."

"So, it's just spina bifida?"

"Ah . . . yeah."

"Oh, thank God!" I said.

Dr. Turnquest-Wells looked at me like I was nuts.

"They had me flat terrified coming in here," I explained. "They told me my baby had no lungs. They said maybe she had a herniated diaphragm— half of those babies die. But I know people with spina bifida, and they grow up, and they have lives, and you just don't know what a relief this is to me!"

"Oh. . . . Okay," she said. She looked carefully at my husband.

I could tell she was thinking perhaps I didn't get it; somehow I had missed that my child would be born with a serious birth defect—and spina bifida is certainly serious. It's a malformation of the spine that causes damage to the spinal nerves, and like any other spinal injury it can result in paraplegia, urinary and bowel control problems, and myriad other chronic health issues. But people with spina bifida usually live and most have normal intelligence.

When we left, Dr. Turnquest-Wells gave me a sepia-toned portrait, three-quarter view, of my baby with her fist in her mouth. I felt as though a great weight had been lifted from my heart and a pall had withdrawn from my eyes. I would not have to bury my baby.

We named her "Cora," after the young woman in James Fenimore Cooper's novel, *The Last of the Mohicans.* Our research revealed that Fenimore Cooper coined the name and that before his novel Cora was not used as a woman's name. Today, it has fallen out of favor and is considered old-fashioned by most. But my husband and I liked the name, and we bestowed it on our unborn girl.

There were more doctors to see. Cora would have to be born at a specialty medical center far from home, and we chose Indiana University Medical Center in Indianapolis. Cora would need two surgeries shortly after birth; these would be done at adjacent Riley Hospital for Children. Cora's delivery, by Caesarian section, would be performed by Dr. Lillie Mae Padilla, a small, reassuringly energetic obstetrician and perinatologist, whose native language was Spanish.

Dr. Padilla examined me and Cora in another marathon ultrasound session, which we drove through a blizzard to get to. Partway through the exam, Dr. Padilla said, "I hate to keep saying 'the baby, the baby.' Does she have a name?"

"Her name is Cora," I said.

"Heart," said Dr. Padilla. When I frowned, she said, "Cora means 'heart' in Spanish. It's a woman's nickname, short for 'Corazon.'"

So, we were wrong about Fenimore Cooper coining the name, but right about the name itself. She is Cora, our dear little heart.

Cora was born on May first—May Day. Six weeks later, Dr. Wigginton—the one who first knew my baby had a problem—gives me a commemorative spoon. "I just wanted you to have a perfect baby," he says.

I think of Cora: Cora, who spent twelve days in neonatal intensive care. Who came through three surgeries in her first two days of life. Who may or may not walk; who may or may not have full control of her bowels. Who may or may not be a doctor, a musician, a bookworm, a dog trainer, or a gardener. Who may be tall or short, pretty or homely, generous or stingy, vivacious or taciturn. It is too soon to know. Just like it would be too soon to know these things with any other baby. Who can say what Cora might do, how she might be?

Later, when Cora is with me, I see my doctor out in public. We walk over to say hello, Cora and I, she with her bright blue eyes and rosebud mouth, I with my heart on my sleeve and in my arms.

"I want you to meet someone," I say, holding her up. "This is Cora. She's my perfect baby."

—*Jennifer Busick*

When He Is New

At such an altitude, the blue drains away. The color of the sky seems to seep backward toward heaven. From this slit of a window that I have to bend down to look out of, there is no horizon limiting my view. There is no tree branch, no swarm of gnats, no crow on a telephone wire grounding my thoughts.

My son stirs in his sleep; already one airline seat is too small for his sleeping body. My husband's eyelids flicker but do not open. His neck will be stiff within the half hour. I pass my hand across my belly. It is a few weeks too early to detect movement, still I want our next child to know the feel of my hand from the very beginning.

I watch my husband, Keith, as he sleeps. Imagine if I could kiss his cheek at that moment how nice it would be. How the feel of his skin against my lips would be the same as it has been for the last thirteen years, warm and intoxicating. If there were no other passengers, no belly to maneuver over, no sleeping limbs of an eighteen-month-old sprawled across my lap, I would fall against his cheek and nap. Instead, my eyes wander to my son.

When he sleeps, Mason is most beautiful. His features take on an added fullness, especially around his eyes and lips. He is not what I'd expected. I thought he'd be half me, half his father. But he is all himself. Not a replica of anything. Convinced that all my children would be girls, it is not until he comes out that I realize gender is such an inadequate measure of character. A footnote. Less descriptive than the spacing between his eyelashes, the curve of his baby toe. As if dressing him in blue gives strangers useful information.

No one has ever seemed as wise as he did, that first time he looked up at me, his eyes pinning the swallow against my throat. *I have found you again*, he seemed to say, as if he knew me from some time before. Or perhaps his wisdom is in that moment, having no before or after, nothing to clutter his request, to deter his wanting. *Feed me and I will be yours*, he seemed to demand. He began to suck as if his life depended on it, and he became mine.

As he nursed, his head turned to the side and I discovered his ears. I followed with my finger along the extra fold of each ear, like an intricate maze leading down to his eardrum. In comparison, other human ears are like doughnuts that have been stepped on. What will he listen for, that a flat-eared person doesn't? A group of pediatricians came to look at them. They told us that someone in one of our families must have ears like this. They have been inherited from someone along the line. How many decades has this child's hearing journeyed through? I wonder. What does he know? I watched him for clues, thinking some sign might reveal their purpose.

When he was new, everything else resembled him. A salamander, the letter G on the cover of a library book, a moth. The slightest display of vulnerability in any living thing sent me with tears streaming into Mason's room toward his crib. When he was awake, I worried he should sleep, and when he slept I fought the urge to wake him. I could not concentrate on conversations. He demanded all my attention, even while I slept.

Gradually, I regained my former self and stopped crying at the sight of an injured caterpillar or the parched dirt around a neglected houseplant. I grew accustomed to his breathing, although still it sounded miraculous. After his ears, I studied his hands, so much like his father's.

I watch them now, high above the earth, as his fingers curl toward his palm. If I could burrow my way inside his skin, still I wouldn't be too close. Later, when he is older, I will tell him and the new one, who will turn out to be a shiny bowling ball of a girl, that I loved them both from the beginning. Not the moment I first saw them. Not at the sound of their first cries. Not even when I felt that first turn in my belly. No, love builds more slowly than that. Love begins before we know each place to put it.

I've loved them both since the moment their father smiled my way. From the moment I first eyed the ocean, first tasted pomegranates. From that first day my mother held me in her arms. Love stretches backward, rolls forward, and when it finds its mark, unfolds in every direction, like the sky, like heaven.

—*Pauline Knaeble Williams*

Love Lost and Found

My mother is thirty-nine years old. She has died from cancer. Before she died, she was heartbroken, knowing she had to leave her six children behind.

I am four years old, her youngest child. I am alone. I no longer have a mother and I yearn for her love.

My father works or is at the bar. When he is home, many times he is drunk. There is a lot of yelling and hitting. He is not handling my mother's death very well or the responsibilities of raising young children. Work and drink are his escapes.

I am eight years old. My father has remarried. My sister and I move to a new house, his new wife's house. My older siblings have moved out on their own. My stepmother seems to resent that he brought kids to the marriage with him and that we are not quiet, fastidious, and invisible. We try to be very quiet and to do as we are told, but we seem to irritate her no matter what we do. She is a screamer, and she takes her anger out on us.

My father still drinks. They fight and there is a lot of yelling. My stepmother does not want my sister and me. We walk on eggshells. She calls us "scum." They send us away to live with relatives. I am ten years old. We live with an aunt and uncle. My uncle corners my sister, now an adolescent. She "makes trouble," tells what happens. They send us back to my father and his wife.

I am thirteen. My father does not want my sister and me. We interfere with his life, with his marriage. They send us to live with other relatives, and then with friends, and then a foster home.

I am sixteen, back living with my father and his wife. They still fight; there is still anger and resentment. They kick my sister out of the house. They send me to live with my brother and his wife. They are kind but young and struggling themselves. I am grateful and try not to cause trouble.

I am eighteen. I can start my own new life and leave it all behind. I am smart. I am tough as nails. The chip on my shoulder is my defense, my strength. I love it. I use it. It is my best friend. I go to school and work. I am very functional. I am a survivor.

I protect myself, keep to myself. I had to close

myself off when I was a child or suffer even more. I had to close myself off as an adult because I'd learned that emotions were a weakness. I had no room for weakness. If someone cried, I scoffed. If someone felt sad or depressed, I lost respect. They were weak. I was strong.

Why should my feelings, my emotions be in the open? I did not want pity. No one could give me a mother. No one could love me like a mother. I am an adult now. I cannot change the past. I cannot change my mother's death, leaving young children and an alcoholic, selfish father to manage the mess.

Grow up and live your life the best you can. Shove away the memories of loss and loneliness, the hope for a mother's love. That is what I did.

I am twenty-two, twenty-four, twenty-eight, thirty years old. I am an adult. I am struggling with myself. I have missed the most important thing a child can have: the love of a mother.

I force myself to examine what I carry inside of me. It is very painful but necessary. I realize I will never be normal on the inside. I will carry this sadness and loneliness forever. I accept that. I admit it to myself. I feel at peace with myself. I am more willing to let others see inside of me.

I meet a man. He is kind, and I come to trust him. I tell him everything. He tells me he loves me. He loves me because of my life, in spite of my life.

His compassion exceeds all bounds. He wants to marry me. I become his wife, and he becomes the first family I ever had.

I am thirty-four years old. I am pregnant. I am terrified. I am not a complete person. How can I be a mother? I never had one. How can I love a child? I was not loved as a child. What am I doing? Who am I kidding? I do not know what it means to be a mother. I do not know what it means to be a child. It is not my fault. I just do not know.

How will I know how to love my child? I worry constantly during my pregnancy. I am very insecure and plagued by self-doubt. How will I know what to do? How will I know how to give comfort and love to a baby, a child? I am one of those people who should not have children.

My baby, my son, is born. I am alone with him for the first time. I hold him and give him my breast. No one is there to see. I am alone in the hospital room with him. It is midnight. I help him latch on to my breast to eat. He starts to suckle, so gently, and my body responds by giving him milk. He holds his tiny hands by his face, and I stare at him in wonderment. I talk to him softly and caress his tiny head. It feels so natural holding him in my arms. My heart fills with tender, pure, warm love for him. Something has just changed.

I am thirty-nine years old. I am a mother and I am alive.

My son is four years old. He has a mother who loves him every second of every day.

His father works and comes home to us. There is no yelling or hitting. His father is not drunk. There is love and laughter. We are a family.

The birth of my son has given me what I had yearned for all of my life. It has given me a mother's love. I receive from him a love that is given only to a mother. Through loving him, I now know my mother's love for me. It is full in me. I no longer yearn for a mother; I no longer have that need. I am a mother now, and I am complete.

—*Ellen Cullen*

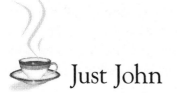 Just John

Before our son was born, my husband and I had a list of interesting names for him. None had any overriding swaying power for either one of us, so we decided to wait until he made his entrance and "call him as we see him." Meanwhile, I secretly entertained exotic combinations of features for my fetal son—he would have golden brown skin, green eyes like his dad but almond-shaped like mine, and luscious loops of curly dark hair.

I was nothing short of stunned when our very ordinary-looking, beige-skinned, brown-eyed, brown-haired newborn son made his earthly debut to the tune of *The Nanny* (the television was on in the birthing room). So certain had I been that he would be the extraordinary beauty our daughter is, I could only stare as he wailed uncharmingly and urinated on the nurse.

All the lovely and lyrical names I had sung to myself while patting my swollen belly flew out of my head. This was no Vincenzio. This wasn't even an Avery—my favorite (and my husband's least favorite) name. This was . . . John.

Yep, John. As average as the child himself. Not average in the ho-hum way, mind you. Children of immigrant grandparents that my husband and I are, for us to have an average baby after an average pregnancy in an above-average hospital in Manhattan— well, isn't that what our grandparents braved the seas for? What could be more American than John? At the time, the world was mourning the beloved John Kennedy Jr.—not a bad namesake for your average American boy. And, for all of them out there, I personally have never met a mean John. And we could always jokingly tell people that we named him John because the first thing he did was "go to the john" immediately upon his exit from the womb and on the less-than-amused nurse.

John. I liked it.

As the drugs wore off and I was able to hold my son, I found myself falling in love, and just thinking. "John" had been on my list. In fact, for a while, it was my first choice. But there is no one in either of our families named John. So why was it on my list from the beginning and why was it the name I actually chose in the end? Then, in one of those moments of clarity that writers love to write about, I remembered.

It was a warm and pleasant summer afternoon in the late 1970s. I was about eleven years old and had discovered my mom's personal library of young adult books. Mom had wanted to become a nurse before her heart murmur prevented it, and as a girl she had a whole collection of books about nurses and medicine. I had already read all about Cherry Ames and had begun reading Sue Barton, visiting nurse. I was fascinated. The beautiful Sue sort of looked like Mom—red hair, fair complexion, fine features. But I especially liked this volume, because her territory was the Lower East Side of Manhattan, where we lived. I enjoyed reading the names of familiar streets in the story—Henry Street, Mott Street, Orchard Street. It made me feel somehow connected to my mom, like I was getting a glimpse of what her life must have been like when she was my age in the 1950s on the Lower East Side.

A slew of aunts and younger cousins had come over for a visit and eventually wanted to go outside to enjoy the day. I was the oldest cousin, too mature to horse around with the others, but too young to do much of anything else in the projects where we lived. Usually, I would stay behind, watching TV; I also loved watching old syndicated shows that I thought my mom might have watched when she was my age.

I pictured her frolicking at a beach party or bopping to do-wop while giggling with her girlfriends, like the girls on the old reruns did.

But that day, for no discernable reason, I decided to join my family and enjoy the end of summer. I took Sue Barton with me. They chose a spot near the edge of the apartment complex where there were two long rows of benches, back to back. My brother, sister, and cousins enjoyed running back and forth between the rows and climbing from bench to bench. They laughed loudly, all five of them, while my mom chatted with her sisters in Spanglish. I sat sideways on one of the benches, looking out toward the Woolworth Tower. I settled into a cross-legged position and buried myself in my book while my cousins clambered around me.

My reading came to an abrupt halt when I came upon a passage that described the fair Sue dealing with the "oppressed Negro children." The phrase jolted me, because we called African-Americans "black" people. I didn't really understand the "oppression" part, but I understood enough to realize that the author saw Sue's visits as the only ray of sunshine in these "Negro children's" otherwise miserable lives. It was as though the author were saying, "How noble of Sue Barton to even care." The tone of the passage was so racist and condescending that I had to reread it several times over, all the while thinking, "That's my mom they're talking about.

That's me they're talking about." For the first time, it dawned on me that the glorified life I had envisioned my mom leading was far from how she actually lived. And even farther from how she was perceived.

If I had been alive then, I wouldn't have been able go to a sock hop or to the same school with white kids. Or even drink from the same water fountain. Or I could be lynched—for trumped-up "crimes" or just for sport. I was engrossed in imagining more and more horrific images, wallowing in my newfound betrayal, when the voice of my three-year-old cousin, Edwin, snapped me out of it.

"Hello!" Edwin called out.

I looked up. Sitting not more than three feet from me on the bench was an elderly gentleman. He was well-dressed, very tall, and at least seventy years old. My cousin had crawled up beside him, inches from his face, to examine this kindly stranger.

"Hello," said the man. "What's your name?"

"Edwin," said my cousin proudly. He scooted even closer to the man. Pointing a tiny finger, he asked, "What's your name?"

"My name is John."

"Don?" Edwin couldn't pronounce the "J" yet.

He nodded deliberately, maybe solemnly. "Yes. John."

"Hello, John!" With that, Edwin climbed around John and continued to play.

No one else had noticed the interaction, but I looked on after my cousin resumed his play. This man, John, was American, judging by the way he spoke. And he was white. He had been born way before the imagined Sue Barton would have been. Even if he hadn't been born in America, he had undoubtedly seen a lifetime of drama—two World Wars, a scientific revolution, and much civil unrest. He had actually seen that era of racial inequality in history, and yet here he was, a well-dressed white man in the United States, sitting amidst these happy brown children who didn't think twice about swinging past and over him in their play. Or pointing an innocent finger in his direction. Or striking up a conversation. Or looking him in the eye. A mere generation before, in some parts of this very country, my country, this would have been unthinkable. And only a few years before that, it could have cost my cousin his life. And this old white man, John, had been alive during it all.

There were plenty of other benches he could have chosen, but he chose this one. I watched as he sat on that bench, facing the Twin Towers, in the projects on the Lower East Side of Manhattan. For all that he must have seen in his lifetime, this man exuded such a calm, contented, and generally good aura that I smiled. Suddenly, I was able to put my relatively short life into perspective as well as my mother's. I silently thanked her for saving her favorite books for me and for allowing me to daydream my afternoons away to reruns of *Bewitched*. I felt lucky—fortunate to have been born and raised in a different era.

I returned to my book. When I looked up a moment later, he was gone, and I felt a little sad.

I've thought of the man on the park bench often throughout my life, wondering who he was and if he were still alive.

I've never forgotten the tranquil feeling I got when I saw him, at such a critical moment in my adolescence. I hoped that, whatever life might bring me, toward the end of it I could sit on a bench of my choosing, surrounded by children, and be happy.

On August 16, 1999, when I gave birth to my baby boy, that is what I hoped for him too. So I named him John. John Avery, to be exact. As it turns out, there are very few children in his generation named John.

Funny how the unassuming becomes remarkable as time goes by.

—*Diana Díaz*

The Expecting
Mother vs.
the Accepting Sibling

I'm here with Mommy to check my baby," says my son, proudly revealing my pregnant belly to the receptionist.

She smiles at her familiar little friend. "Hi, J.P. Midwife Anne will be right with you … and Mommy."

"But Anne has to wait until Daddy gets here. He's coming from work."

"Okay, honey. I'll let her know."

J.P. picks up a Dr. Seuss book from a basket and sits next to me, gently placing his head on my tummy. "Mommy, we want you to read us this book."

For thirty-eight weeks J.P. has been talking "we" talk. We want oatmeal for breakfast. We want to take a walk. We want you to read to us. The eerie part is that my husband and I had never said anything to J.P. about our decision to have another child. Yet, two mornings after we had started our baby-making process, J.P. lifted up my shirt, kissed my tummy, and spoke "we" talk from that moment on.

"Mommy? When will Sarkist come out of your tummy?" asks J.P., no longer interested in the story.

"In another couple of weeks or so."

"But I want Sarkist to come out and play now."

"I think the baby is awake," I say. "Try playing your special game."

J.P. gently presses on my tummy. A moment later the baby inside responds with a kick. J.P. giggles. He presses again. The baby kicks back. J.P. laughs.

"Mommy, will we call my baby Sarkist after it's born?"

"Sarkist will be the baby's nickname."

"Oh, that's right." J.P. puts his mouth close to my tummy. "Hi, Sarkist. That's your nickname. It means 'sweet one' in Ar . . . Ar . . ."

"Armenian."

J.P. waves me off. "I know, I know. Armenian. We'll give you another name when you come out and tell us if you're a boy or a girl."

"J.P.," calls the nurse, "time to check your baby."

J.P. stands in protest. "But Daddy's not here yet."

"How about we get Mommy started, and we'll send Daddy in as soon as he gets here," she suggests.

"Okay." J.P. grabs my hand. "Come on, Mommy. Time to see how big Sarkist is."

I allow him to lead me into the examination room, amazed at how quickly the last three years have passed. It seems like just yesterday I was pregnant with this little boy and filled with the same anxious excitement about his impending arrival that he now displays for "his" baby.

I step onto the scale.

"Expectant siblings first," says the nurse.

"Oh, right. My mistake." I step down.

J.P. hops up onto the scale, then strains to see the nurse move the weights.

"Just perfect," she says. "Now let's give Mommy a turn."

As she weighs me and I answer the usual pre-exam questions, J.P. pretends the office stool is a steering wheel and drives around the small room. This is the only diversion he ever allows himself during our midwife appointments, because he's always eager to get back to the business at hand.

"When do we get to hear my baby's heartbeat?"

"Just as soon as Anne and Daddy come."

"Did someone say Daddy?" asks my husband, entering with our midwife.

While J.P. fills them in on our appointment thus far, I can't help but wonder how J.P.'s excitement at being an expectant sibling will translate into actually becoming a big brother. How will he handle it when Sarkist is no longer an abstract concept with a nickname contained in Mommy's tummy, but rather a crying "thing" demanding attention from the two people who, up until that point, gave J.P. their single-minded focus?

My own brother is three years older than I am and by all accounts was quite doting upon my arrival home from the hospital. After I learned to walk, talk, and grab toys, however, we entered the tumultuous world of sibling rivalry that thirty years later we are just beginning to navigate with any sense of decorum.

That, of course, leads to my own self-doubts. Do I have enough love to give to two children? How can I possibly love this second child as much as I love my first? How do I go about making both my children feel equally yet uniquely loved? Will J.P. get angry if he hears me lull the baby to sleep with the same songs I used to sing to him? Will he still feel love for "his baby" when that child cries us all awake at 2:00 A.M. for a feeding? Will J.P. feel abandoned when I don't let him have a midnight snack too?

I've heard it said that demanding a child to accept a new sibling is like a husband expecting his spouse to accept another wife in their home. Admittedly, as much as I love my husband and trust our relationship, I would not be at all thrilled if he came home one day and said, "Honey, meet our new wife."

"Don't hurt my baby!" yells J.P., waking me from my thoughts.

"It's okay," I comfort. "You've seen Anne do this

before. She's just pressing on my tummy to determine what position Sarkist is in."

"That doesn't hurt my baby?"

"Not at all. Anne knows what she's doing and is very gentle. It's just like when you play your game with Sarkist."

"Perhaps it's time to put jelly on the belly," Anne suggests.

"Jelly on the belly! Jelly on the belly!" J.P. sings happily, anticipating his favorite part of these checkups. Anne lets him help squirt the ultrasound gel on my stomach and turn on the heart machine. *Whoosh, whoosh, whoosh, whoosh.*

"Hear that, Mommy? That's my baby's heartbeat!" J.P. puts my hand on his chest. "Feel that, Mommy? That's my heartbeat. Sarkist and I have the same heart. Whoosh, whoosh, whoosh, whoosh."

Suddenly, I am reminded of a conversation I had with a Native American medicine woman during my first trimester.

"It's the wildest thing," I had confided to Grandmother Mechi. "Not only is J.P. overprotective of the baby growing inside me, but he knew I was pregnant even before I knew."

"That means your son and your baby knew each other in another life," Grandmother Mechi had replied. "They are happy to be reuniting in this one. They will always have a close connection."

I watch J.P. help clear the gel off my abdomen.

"There you go, Sarkist, all clean. When you come out, I'll help Mommy give you a bath and feed you and change you."

"I've never seen a little boy so excited about becoming a big brother. Your baby sure picked the right family," says Anne.

"And I picked the right baby," J.P. replies. "Sarkist and I are going to grow up to be best friends."

Then, it hits me. I have been given a wonderful gift—a little boy with instinctive and unconditional love for "his" baby. J.P. doesn't question what will come next, because he only cares about right now. Rather than worry about the future, I, too, will nurture the present. I will stop obsessing about "what if" and start focusing on "what is." I will keep in mind that although I am about to become a mother for the second time, I am still a first-time mother to J.P. I will handle each new sibling-rivalry challenge that might occur the same way I've handled every other new event for the past three years—as it comes. Accepting, instead of expecting.

—*Judy L. Adourian*

All He Will Need

I have never approached any event in my life anticipating defeat. I have always been a planner, always believed that with the right angle and appropriate amount of persistence, success would be mine … until I found myself in labor with my first child.

In that brief but blinding moment when even your own body fails to follow orders, where nothing runs to plan and all of life becomes a series of gasping breaths and nothing more, I began to doubt my ability for success. After all, in the middle of that monumental effort, I had still another epiphany: I was eighteen years old, unmarried, and had nothing to offer a child. What was I doing in a labor ward?

"I can't do this!" I yelled. A declaration seemed appropriate at the time.

"Of course you can," said the very efficient, very patient midwife. She chuckled softly while she stroked the hair back from my forehead. "This is transition. At this point, everyone feels they can't do this, but you can. Women have been doing this for eons, and they'll be doing it a long time after. I think you're as good as any of them."

"This is not a transition," I sobbed, partly at her misplaced faith and partly at my horrible realization. "This is my life!"

This same midwife had conducted my antenatal classes, the ones for teenaged parents. There was no doubt she understood exactly what I meant. So I believe she spoke truthfully when she tutted, sat on the edge of my bed, took my hand in hers, and said, "That it is, sweetheart. You've picked a hard road, I'll grant you that, but I think you're up to it. Now is not the time for doubt. Now is the time to believe … in yourself and in miracles. You're producing one right now, you know."

Gathering up my strength and what little faith I had left in myself, I clung to her hand and her compassion, and cried until my little miracle appeared.

I named him Patrick and watched him sleep quietly in his crib beside my bed for two days. On the third day of our stay, doubt and fear again overwhelmed me. That morning, my infant son began to cry. I held him, I cooed to him, I fed him, and, weeping, I pleaded with him to stop. Eventually, the crying ceased, his and mine, but I was left feeling inadequate and desperate. Again, I feared I might fail. This time, my fear was not for me but for my Patrick.

My midwife reappeared that day too. In her cool blue uniform and with her unwavering eyes, she sat, the way women do, one hip on, one hip off the edge of my bed. "I hear you're not feeling so great today."

"I have nothing to give him," my voice quavered and broke on the words. Tears burned hot in my eyes. "No father, no family, not even a real home."

Perhaps I was being a little hysterical; they say the baby blues will do that to a person. I did have a family who would love us, help us, and house us, but it was not what I'd envisioned. I'd dreamed that my first child would arrive home to the arms of a besotted father, a white picket fence, and a swing on the tree in the backyard. Shattered dreams have sharp edges, and they snagged and scratched at my throat as I swallowed my reality.

My midwife was not the least bit phased by the rising catch in my voice. She gently asked, "Did you not think about this before? Did no one ask you what you had to offer a child?"

"Yes," I gulped like a child who'd scraped her knee climbing the forbidden tree and now was having it bandaged.

"And what did you tell them?"

"That I could give him all my love and caring. I would give him all my heart."

"That, little mother, is all he will ever need."

She was right. For fourteen years, Patrick has lived in my heart—filling me with joy and purpose. For fourteen years, Patrick has blossomed in the fertile soil of a mother's love. And for the love of Patrick, I was spurred to great feats.

While Patrick was small, I pursued and received a degree in education. Later, while I was teaching school to support us, I went on to earn my master's. In the process, I attended preschool Christmas pageants and remembered dental appointments. Scrubbed vomit from carpet and removed ink from walls. Read stories and kicked soccer balls. Kissed owies and gave time-outs. And loved my boy.

Now that Patrick is a teenager, I encourage him to choose his own path and find his own solutions to problems. I remind him to believe in himself and that I believe in him. I teach him the virtues of persistence and that blessings sometimes come disguised as obstacles. I challenge him not to allow fear to defeat or diminish him, and I assure him that miracles do happen.

Most important, I tell him and show him, every day, that I love him. Because now I know it is all he will ever need.

Giving life gave me the need and the motivation to make a life, a good life, for my son and myself. Of course, there has been plenty of rain along with the sunshine, and there have been missteps as well as successes. But I have laughed more than I have cried, and I wouldn't trade the life I've shared with my son for anything. Because loving Patrick is all I really need, too.

—Rebecca Bloomer

High Fives All Around

While pregnant with my first child, I fielded countless comments from friends, acquaintances, and strangers. Some were funny, like when a young male colleague said to me as I left work for maternity leave, "Well, good luck with the fetus." (The fetus?) Some were annoying: "You're so small for twenty weeks." (The woman who said this probably meant it as a compliment, but it made me feel like I would give birth to a raisin.) Some were odd, like when a young woman saw me waddling along at thirty weeks and asked, "Do you have a limp?" And some were just lame: "Looks like you and your hubby had some fun!" (Wink, wink.)

But the comments that really touched my nerves were about childbirth. I was already scared enough about labor; hearing other people's horrific tales didn't help.

"When my Sara was born, I thought I was going to die," a woman confided to me at the doctor's office. "She broke my tailbone and nearly split me in two. My eyes were bloodshot for a week." A broken tailbone? Split in two? Eyes bloodshot for a week? This did little to calm my nerves. Soon after, a friend at work told me, "I hardly ever swear, but getting that baby out hurt so badly, I swore like a sailor."

Would I be a bloody, foul-mouthed, bloodshot, split-in-two mess? Would my baby come out unharmed? Could I do it?

Then there was the video I saw in my birthing class, which was supposed to prepare me for labor but only served to ramp up my fears. It portrayed one woman in prelabor, rocking primly with pursed lips in a rocking chair, as if determined not to let the experience get the best of her, and another woman in labor, moaning and hollering while attempting to focus on a picture of her dog. Neither portrayal allayed my fears. Nor did the nurse who taught the class, who said we should feel free to scream like wild animals if we felt so inclined.

Would labor possibly turn me into a wild animal? A froth-mouthed lioness? It all seemed so freaky and scary.

My mom's memories of labor, in contrast, were comforting, but so vague and lovely that I hardly trusted them. "I remember the warm towels the nurses wrapped you in right after you were born," she said, "and how beautiful you were. I knew I wanted to have another baby right away."

So my labor fears stayed with me as my belly grew, and my strange, graphic dreams continued. I dreamt of birthing a bat-like creature, of having a pregnant belly that looked like an over-cooked muffin, and of careening, fully pregnant, down swervy waterslides. I remembered, for the first time in years, how horrified I'd been in kindergarten class after watching a vivid movie of a woman giving birth, and how I could hardly stand to look at the cabbage rolls in tomato sauce my mom had made for dinner that night.

Then one day a friend, who wasn't even pregnant, said a simple thing that helped to calm me: "One way or another, you'll get through it. It won't go on forever."

True, I thought, *no matter what, the hard part of labor will last no more than a day, if that.* And I thought of all the rowing, swimming, running, and triathlon races I'd endured. I decided I would mentally prepare for labor like I would an athletic event. Maybe I'd even drink a lot of water and eat an energy bar as soon as the contractions began. I would breathe, focus, push through it, embrace it even, and know that at some point, no matter what, I'd make it to the finish line.

I remembered a conversation I'd had years earlier with a friend in college, over pie and tea, about enduring pain. My friend had asked how my rowing workouts were going, knowing that in the middle of a timed ergometer workout, I had suddenly let go of the handle. My leg muscles were burning and my lungs ached, so I'd just stopped, without meaning to.

"Well," I'd said, "I've figured out how to push through the pain and not be scared of it." She eyed me suspiciously, but I continued. "I just keep pushing with my legs and pulling with my arms, and I embrace the pain and let it hurt. I don't fight it. I let the pain wash over me, and then it's almost a good feeling." My friend's eyes grew wide. I'm sure she expected to hear a chatty answer to a casual question, not a dissertation on pain. What came out of my mouth sounded kind of cliché, yet it was exciting and real to me. Empowering. I could do anything. I was strong.

I had forgotten about that conversation, because I hadn't pushed myself to that extent in an athletic event for years. But now, a few weeks from my due date, I remembered. *Labor*, I thought, *will be the greatest athletic event of my life. I will let it happen. I'll feel it.*

Maybe I'd purse my lips like the woman in the video. Maybe I'd scream like a wild animal. Maybe I'd demand drugs. Who knew? But one way or another, I'd get through it.

And I did. Three weeks later, my water broke and the twenty-one-hour marathon began. To my surprise, my body took over, and I just hung on. The contractions came slowly and mildly at first, and then faster and stronger, rolling through me again and again and again. It took all my strength and willpower to stay focused, to make it to the finish line and push the baby out, but I did it. I did it! And no medals or trophies I'd won in the past could begin to compare to this grand reward—my newborn baby girl, with her penetrating eyes, nibbly toes, and snuffly breath.

Yes, labor was more painful and frightening than any rowing race had ever been. And yes, I'd panted, groaned, and even screamed like a split pig (as my husband put it). But when the doctor plopped my daughter's squirming, wet body on my chest and I kissed her silky hair, I was overcome with gratitude and joy, buzzed in the zone between elation and exhaustion. Any amount of pain and effort was worth that feeling—a feeling of unparalleled honor in having created and birthed a life. The empowerment I felt post-labor was much greater than anything I'd ever felt before.

Hours later, while looking at my sleeping baby in the hospital bassinet, still achy and spent but happy, I reveled in my newfound knowledge: I am wondrously connected to all mothers everywhere, throughout the world and throughout time. We are strong. We all did it.

High fives all around.

—Gretchen Maurer

 Waiting

We waited to have kids. Well, I waited. I wanted to play first, have a career, and squirrel away some money. Wait for the right moment, I told myself. Live a little and be ready for kids. As it turns out, the right moment doesn't exist, and things don't always happen by the book. You can wait a lifetime, but pregnancy arrives when it does—ready or not.

I married a wonderful man in college, but neither of us felt we were ready for kids. My husband accepted an engineering job right after graduation, and we packed our bags. We traded fir trees and family in the Pacific Northwest for exhaust fumes and career opportunities in Northern California. Clinging to each other, we created a new life for ourselves as a couple of DINKs—double income, no kids. The years rolled by, and life was good.

Silicon Valley in the 1980s was crammed with fast-lane folks like us. Work hard, play harder: It was our creed and lifestyle choice. Sixty- to seventy-hour work weeks were not uncommon, and we lived for the weekends—sand, sun, and crowded bars. None of our friends had children; in fact, most were single. Stories of ticking biological clocks were legend, fabricated to test the work ethic of dedicated employees and to weed out the weak. Betty Crocker, a minivan, and kids could wait. We enjoyed our twenties with hedonistic zeal, stayed up late, bought expensive toys, and traveled the world. After we'd been happily married for seven child-free years, our parents stopped asking about grandchildren.

When my husband's father became ill, we moved back to the Northwest. Suddenly, being close to family became a priority, so we purchased our first home in Happy Valley, a pleasant suburb of Portland, Oregon. Happy Valley, so cliché it could have been called Mayberry or Walton's Mountain. I marched right out and bought a Crock-Pot, but we still weren't ready for kids. Instead, we bought a dog, a black and white Siberian pup with melt-your-heart chocolate brown eyes and pearly teeth. We named her White Fang.

Many couples, if they are honest, will tell you that owning a dog is good training for family life. Having a dog is a serious commitment; you have to remember to feed the dog, let the dog out to run, and make sure it gets to the vet every once in a while. And good pet ownership is a great deal more. There's potty training, obedience school, and loving discipline when your puppy chews a favorite leather shoe. Take a deep breath and count to ten. You can't take off on a whim when you have a dog, can't fly to Spain for the weekend. A kennel? Not the places we saw. Someone has to care for and love the furry child like a parent would. Someone needs to get up on a Sunday morning at 6:00 A.M. to let the dog out, no matter whether you have an important meeting to get to or a hangover to nurse. At the crack of dawn, sometimes earlier, your dog barks, comes in to lick your face, and you get up—ready or not.

Our life with a dog was good, but different. We settled into our home, I learned how to use the Crock-Pot, and White Fang got straight As in puppy kindergarten. Now, we had married friends and worked slightly fewer hours. We were thirty-something and living in the suburbs, but still no kids in sight. When my younger sister and her husband announced they were pregnant, the family cheered and I thought I heard a slight *tick, tick*.

One morning I woke up to some serious ticking. It wasn't a soft sound, like the hall clock I remember lulling me to sleep at Grandma's house. This was a loud noise that filled my head, crashing like surf in my ears: *tick, tick, tick.* I was slightly alarmed, but it stopped once I got to work.

Then, my sister had her baby on Christmas Eve. The whole clan gathered at the hospital with presents, a potluck dinner, and a bottle of champagne to celebrate the newest member of the family. He was cute as a button, swaddled up sleeping in my sister's arms. And it started again, even louder this time: *tick, tick, tick, tick!* And it didn't stop when we went home. From then on, at any time and in any place, it would start up again: *tick, tick, tick, tick* . . . .

We didn't wait much longer. How could we, with all that ticking going on in my head? Not long after my thirty-fifth birthday I was pregnant, and nine months later I delivered a beautiful, healthy baby boy. We thought that, as a newborn, he looked more like Winston Churchill than like either of us, but we were still thrilled. He was our very own, and we loved him more than words.

When we arrived home from the hospital, our dog made a careful inspection of the new arrival. She poked her wet nose again and again into his diaper, giving him a detailed sniff. Finally, White Fang welcomed my son into our family pack with a lick on the cheek.

Just one year later, I was pregnant again. But this time was different.

A routine trip to the OB/GYN turned our lives inside-out. A blood test for AFP, a protein found in the fluid surrounding the baby during pregnancy, had come back with abnormal results. I listened with my heart in my throat as the doctor explained that abnormal alpha-fetoprotein levels could indicate a neural tube defect, such as spina bifida, chromosomal abnormalities, birth defects, or Down syndrome. More tests would be required. On cue, a lab assistant rolled an ultrasound machine into the room and squirted massive blobs of ice cold jelly onto my stomach. The doctor flipped on a switch and rolled the handheld transducer around my tummy like a small iron. "Hmmm . . . " she said, forehead wrinkled as she stared at the screen. The machine swished and bleeped, making curious noises while the doctor moved her hand around my slick and swollen belly. She printed pictures and made notations in my chart, but didn't say a thing.

Birth defect? "How could this be possible?" I asked the doctor. I was doing everything by the book: eating my dark-leafy green vegetables, choking down quarts of milk, and staying away from booze, secondhand smoke, and anything I would have done in my twenties.

"Well," she answered, "You waited a little too long to have kids. Generally, women over the age of thirty-five are at increased risk of complications, including birth defects, chromosome abnormalities, and miscarriage."

I didn't hear much after that, because my head was buzzing, but I think the doctor explained the test and what she called my "options." For the next hour, I was lost in a fog of medical terms, simply nodding along with a forced sense of calm. I had the urge to vomit, but managed to hold off until I reached the parking lot outside the doctor's office.

When I got home, there was already a message on the answering machine. An amniocentesis had been scheduled as well as an appointment with a genetic counselor. I was to call the office if I had any questions. Instead, I phoned my husband at work and prayed I could talk to him without dissolving into a weepy mess.

"Honey, don't worry," he assured me. "We'll get through this together."

The amniocentesis procedure is not for the faint of heart. A long, thin needle is inserted into the abdomen, piercing through layers of fat and muscle tissue and into the baby's amniotic sac. Then, a small amount of fluid is drawn out, and the fetal cells in it are examined. I was told this test was needed to rule out the condition that was feared in my case: Down syndrome.

Fear clenched my jaw as I lay waiting on the table, my belly naked and exposed, a red stripe painted below my flattened bellybutton, and the pungent smell of Betadine hanging in the air.

"Just try to relax," the doctor said. "You'll feel a little pinch." What this means is, "Brace yourself. This is going to hurt like hell!" And it did.

Later, after the test, I had to translate again. "We'll call you as soon as we have the results," actually means, "Go home and try not to think that your baby might have a life-limiting, if not life-threatening, birth defect."

The genetic counseling appointment wasn't fun either, but at least it didn't involve needles. My husband and I were seated in a richly appointed office with leather couches, a Persian rug, and red mahogany furniture. Large boxes of tissues were scattered around the room, obviously for us, so I took a few sheets in preparation.

"Who is our counselor?" my husband asked, trying to break the tension. "Hugh Hefner?" We laughed and waited for someone dressed in a smoking jacket to join us.

The counselor arrived (without jacket) and handed us lengthy health questionnaires. "I'll be back in a bit," she said and left the room.

"Mother's age over 35?" I checked the yes box and asked myself for the millionth time why I had waited all those years. If only I had known . . . my baby . . . That's when I used the tissues. Farther down the page, my husband pointed to another question: "If test results are positive, would you like information about terminating your pregnancy?" Worry painted his face. A silent agreement not to go that route passed between us, but I could not hide my fear or sadness. The tissues came in handy.

When we finished our questionnaires, the counselor joined us to review the answers. We spoke frankly about conditions, complications, and again, options. For almost two hours, it was like a sick version of family disease, history, and disability tic-tac-toe. Then, our answers were carefully noted and documented in a file.

Sometime in the second week of waiting for my amnio results, I noticed that the doctors and nurses stopped smiling. I was going in every few days for an ultrasound to check my fluid levels, but the doctor's office felt cold and clinical. People stopped referring to my baby and started calling it "the fetus." Instead of having a pregnant glow, I now looked "flushed" to the nurses. I wondered whether the staff knew something I didn't.

Preparing for the worst, I waited and prayed each day for the grace of keeping my faith. I prayed for strength in the midst of my fear, and I prayed for the precious gift I carried with me. For three and a half weeks we waited. During that time, I realized that the bond I had developed with my baby was stronger than any test result or diagnosis. I knew that he or she would be born into a wonderful family and that I would be the child's mother. Ready or not.

Thankfully, the test results were normal. Today, my daughter is a vibrant and rambunctious kindergartener. She has wild hair the color of honey and a smile that warms me through. All the worry and wait, frustration and pain were worth it. My kids are worth it. And to this day, neither of them has chewed up a leather shoe.

—Piper Selden

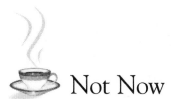 Not Now

Blue. Positive. Pregnant. Definitely pregnant. All three tests confirmed what I already knew, but didn't want to know. The timing was all wrong. I had just received an exciting promotion. My husband and I had recently purchased a new car and a new home, and we were still adjusting to those added expenses. We had a plan, a five-year plan, and becoming parents wasn't in it. Not yet. First, we wanted to reach our respective career goals and save up a nest egg. First, we wanted time alone together as a couple. We wanted to travel. Later, when our marriage, our financial foundation, and our careers were solid, we would start a family. Not now, after only three months as man and wife.

This major kink in our carefully laid plans had not come about because of carelessness. I had been diligent in taking every single birth control pill and in taking them at the same time every day. My mother had warned me that we were a very fertile family. My great-grandmother had had one child in February and another in December of the same year. My mom claimed that the only reason I didn't have two dozen brothers and sisters was Dad's insistence, after the third "pill baby," on having her "tubes tied." She also said my siblings and I were living proof that "the pill" did not cause birth defects. All of us were healthy "brainiacs" who also excelled at various sports. She joked about birth-control-pill babies being "super-babies." My husband would not be amused. After all, this was the man whose response to the stories of fertility in my family was to give me an alarm that reminded me to take my pill at the same time every day. He'd never believed that the women in my family actually took the pill as prescribed. What would he think now?

Wiping away tears, I quickly put the pregnancy tests in a garbage bag and stuffed it under the bathroom sink. If my husband awakened in the middle of the night, I certainly did not want him to see pregnancy tests everywhere. Nor would stumbling across them first thing in the morning be any way to find out that we were unexpectedly expecting. I had to tell him myself, somehow. But first I needed to sort out my own mixed-up emotions. As new and untimely as the pregnancy was, I was already feeling glimmers of what can only be described as motherly love. My overriding emotion, though, was fear of how my husband would react when I told him that, ready or not, we were pregnant.

I thought about writing him a long letter and giving him options: divorce me, change our whole lives around and have the baby, or . . . what? This is not the way I'd thought it would be. I'd envisioned that, when the time was right and we were actually trying to conceive and the miracle happened, I'd leave little clues around the house until he realized we were pregnant. Then, he'd whoop with joy and take me in his arms, telling me how happy he was and how wonderful everything would be, and we'd celebrate our good fortune. I had never pictured sitting alone in the bathroom in the middle of the night, silently weeping and falling apart, trying to keep my pregnancy from my husband until I could come up with a way, and the courage, to break the "bad news."

I pulled myself together and went back to bed, but I just tossed and turned. My mind was going a hundred miles a minute and I couldn't turn it off. When my restlessness roused my husband and he asked what was wrong, I brushed it off by saying I was just stressed about something at work. At least there was some truth to that.

If my calculations were correct, I was one month pregnant. The baby would arrive in eight months—

the start of our busiest season at work. *How much worse could this get?* I wondered, staring at the ceiling, waiting for answers that, like sleep, never came.

Exhausted, I dragged myself to work the next morning and walked around in a daze all day. Fortunately—since many of my coworkers viewed motherhood like a horrific plague that was contagious and could destroy your career—I could attribute my preoccupation to all the changes going on in the company. Every time someone congratulated me on my promotion, I thought, *What are you going to say when you find out I'm pregnant?* I'd seen it before: the pity in other people's eyes when an unplanned pregnancy disrupts a woman's career.

At the end of what had been the longest day of my life, I was glad to go home, but I still dreaded facing my husband. I didn't want to pretend anymore or to fight; I didn't have the energy for either. I was glad to see he was not home yet.

When I walked into the house, I noticed a pink rose on the floor. Then I saw a yellow rose, and then another pink one and another yellow one, and then more, creating a path of alternating pink and yellow roses leading to my favorite chair. On the chair I found three wrapped packages, labeled "1," "2," and "3." I stood there dumbfounded for a moment, wondering whether I'd forgotten the anniversary of our first date or first kiss or some holiday, and then I remembered—my promotion. We hadn't officially celebrated it yet. *What a thoughtful guy*, I thought— and then, *I might as well enjoy this while it lasts, 'cause when he finds out . . .*

I sat down and opened the first note. It read, "I love you heaps. You deserve this and so much more." I opened the package and laughed. Inside was a gift certificate for a pedicure, my favorite indulgence in the whole world. My delight quickly faded, as I told myself that I'd probably need to trade it in for baby products.

On to package number two. The note read, "Being married to you just keeps getting sweeter everyday." I opened a box of my favorite chocolates. Yes! Decadently delicious and ... fattening. *Just what a pregnant woman needs*, I reminded myself bitterly. *If I eat the entire box now, maybe I'll slip into a sugar-induced coma.*

A tear escaped. I tried to enjoy my husband's thoughtful gifts and loving sentiments, but all I could think about was how disappointed he was going to be when he found out that our carefully made plans were destroyed. I didn't even want to open the third package. This was making me feel even guiltier.

I slowly ate one of the chocolates and gathered my courage. The note on the last package read,

"I know your secret. We can celebrate tonight. I love you very much. P.S.—Did you know you can't buy blue roses?"

Blue roses? Why on earth would he want blue roses? My mind raced. Then it hit me. . . . *No. He could not know I'm pregnant. I've been so careful.* My fingers trembled as I opened gift number three. It was a book. As I read the title, I could not believe my eyes: *What to Expect When You're Expecting.*

Was I in the right house? Was I dreaming? I reread the note. He said we could "celebrate" tonight. In that moment, the weight lifted from my shoulders. There would be no divorce, no harsh words, no recriminations. Tonight, we would celebrate . . . and begin making new plans, for our baby.

—Mary Steele Allen

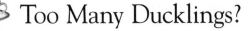 Too Many Ducklings?

It was 8:10 A.M., and I was throwing sandwiches into lunch bags, looking anxiously at my watch. *If the babysitter isn't here in two minutes, I decided, I'll pack up Abraham and take him with us.*

"You forgot to listen to me read last night, Mom. Can I read to you now?" six-year-old Elisha asked.

"Sure, go ahead. Even if I'm not here, just keep going. I'm still listening."

"Anyone seen my shoes?" Isaac, my eight-year-old, yelled.

"Sign my planner, Mom." Noah, eleven, presented his planner in front of my nose as I tossed bags of chips into lunch boxes.

"Don't forget I've got piano right after school, Mom. Please don't be late!" Naphtali, thirteen, urged.

"'Fred . . . gets . . . a . . . duck.' Are you listening, Mom?"

"Fred buys a dog . . . yes, go ahead," I called behind me as I retrieved Abraham, whose foot was stuck in the stair railing.

"No, a duck, Mom!"

"Yes, a duck, an ugly duckling," I repeated. Abraham, fifteen months, was still in his sleeper, and his diaper was soaked through. "Too many ducklings," I muttered, scooping him up and running upstairs to the changing table. I thought of the book by the same title, about a mother duck with ten wayward ducklings, written by some poor man named Quakenbush. I smiled at his name and wondered how he would feel knowing I had adopted his title as my mantra in times of stress. I checked my watch at the top of the stairs.

"Two minutes! We're leaving in two minutes!" I bellowed.

Deciding to skip the diaper change, I set the baby down and ran to the mirror for a quick look, frowned, pulled another layer of red lipstick across my lips, headed down the stairs, and checked the window. The babysitter was still not here. I ran back upstairs, grabbed Abraham, and marched down the stairs and out the front door.

Elisha walked out the door behind me, holding his book in front of his face. "'Let's get another pet,' says Dad . . .'"

"I don't have any shoes!" Isaac shouted at me as I sped past.

"Then go barefoot," I shot back. He misplaced his shoes every day.

"This is it! I'm leaving!" Baby in one arm, briefcase in the other, I strode out into the rain and toward the minivan just as the babysitter pulled into the driveway. I did an about-face, thrust Abraham into the sitter's arms, and sprinted back to the van as the kids spilled out of the house. Isaac ran barefoot, shoes in hand, and dove into the open door of the car.

"Too many ducklings," I sighed again, deeply troubled.

I was two months pregnant. I had just found out the night before, and I could hardly carry the weight of this knowledge. Even amidst the mayhem, a hundred questions were firing in my head, one in particular sounding over and over: Is there really room for one more?

Ten hours earlier, in the bathroom, when the test stick turned blue—a solid blue line cutting across the tiny window like a slash across my life—I could not breathe at first. Then, when I found air, I used it for crying and for great exhalations of disbelief and shock. How could this happen, despite birth control, our too-busy lives, and my husband traveling so often? Even as I ran through all the impossibilities, I felt guilty, as though I were already tainting this being, whoever it was.

I thought of all the other times I had stood in that porcelain courtroom, before the sink and the stick, willing only one verdict: pink, blue, single line, double line, whatever the sign for Yes! I recalled the ecstasy of that moment, when the mysterious reality of what that centimetered mark signified hit home . . . that the life within me, flesh within my own flesh, would soon swell my belly and then come down the chute into the world and my arms and my life. Five times I had done this. And then, with equal joy—glory!—we were done.

I was already anticipating the youngest graduating from the church nursery and then the toddler room. *Imagine,* I thought, *in one more year, I'll walk by these doors triumphant. A survivor! No more infants; no more nursery.* As each child grew steadily toward independence, the exhilaration and exhaustion of those baby years would fade, and I, too, could move onward and upward.

And then, in a single moment, I was back. How could I do this again? How would we find room in our already too-small house? How could I find love for one more? What about my career?

Over the next several weeks, the shock and impossibility of having another baby weighed heavily and constantly on my mind. I tried to simply carry on, fulfilling my duties at work and caring for the children who already filled our house, all the while struggling with the knowledge that I was being called to something I could not do.

At fifteen weeks, I was summoned to the clinic for an ultrasound. I lay back on the table, my shirt under my armpits, my bladder bursting, thinking mostly of the research writing class I would be teaching that night. I hoped it could be done quickly; I had so much to do.

The technician squirted the gel on my belly, adjusted the screen so I could see it, and placed the wand on my abdomen. I'd had several ultrasounds before and knew the routine. I watched the blank screen impassively. Suddenly, it sizzled to life. A tiny child instantly emerged, swimming, flailing, with perfectly formed head, hands, feet, and the last part—yes, a penis. I almost shook my head to clear the screen in my mind that had been blank all these weeks. It's a boy! Transfixed, I watched his acrobatics, all other thoughts gone.

In that moment I remembered that this pregnancy was not merely something happening to my body. This "intruder" was not a passive object—it was so clearly a child. He was already my son. And he was anything but passive! At fifteen weeks, he was already engrossed in his own athletic circuit. *Like my other boys*, I thought, smiling and holding back tears.

I had missed so much! All that time, all those weeks, I'd had so little to do with this baby. In every other pregnancy, I had followed the cell-on-cell creation, the day-by-day development of each child. With books in hand, I'd known exactly when the eyelids formed, when the heart began beating, when the fingernails inched into place. Somehow, I'd felt that I was necessary to each baby's growth, that it was my knowledge and attentiveness, my prayers and desires that fed the tiny body, that made it all happen. Then, when each child was born, I'd held in my arms the one I knew I'd helped create.

Not this time. Fifteen weeks into the pregnancy, and I had no connection with this baby. He was a stranger to me. I had sent him no special thoughts or prayers. Had he been listening, he would have heard nothing from me but worry, nothing but rehearsals of all I could not do. Yet, here he was, the center of spinning blood and spiraling brain passages, the steady beat of heart and flutter of hands and feet—all of it progressing without me.

Then, it struck me: How could I think my attention was required for the precise and perfect formation of every organ and part? How could I believe that it was my own consciousness that kept the miniature feet kicking, the blood pumping, the brain crackling with new energy? I should have known better. I should have remembered the many walks I had taken along the ocean cliffs near my house, with lupine and wild geraniums bursting with color, voles scrabbling along their trails, eagles swirling overhead—all of creation alive, apart from my presence or consciousness. If anything depended upon me alone for the orderly progression and cycling of its molecules, it surely wouldn't survive—like the plants in my house and the garden I sometimes try to grow. Clearly, though, someone is conscious. It is God, of course. It is His wakefulness, His loving attention, that keeps the world humming along—including the new-forming child within my body.

I lay there on the table, belly exposed to the air, watching the baby I knew would be my last, knowing I had been right after all. I was being called to a love I could not find room for. I was being called to what I could not do. But someone else could, and was already doing it, with or without me. And if this Creator could fashion this wondrous child within me, could He not also create in me an equally wondrous love for this child? I already knew the answer.

—*Leslie Leyland Fields*

The Secret Club

ome on in," the woman greeted me. "Welcome." She took my bridal-shower gift and set it on a table with other packages and gift bags—a sumptuous stack of white paper and silver ribbon reminiscent of a wedding cake—then asked, "You're Candace, right?"

"Yes, Robert's wife," I said, knowing I would be the only representative there from the groom's side of the family. I took a steadying breath. *It's just a wedding shower,* I reminded myself as I followed her past a huge, stone fireplace. Deliver the gift, stay a while after the bride-to-be arrives, then leave, duty done.

Being in a strange place and meeting new people didn't usually faze me, but at age forty-one and four months into my fourth pregnancy—the one we prayed would finally result in a baby—I had contracted an acute case of anxiety. We entered a warm kitchen swarming with women. My right hand cupped the slight roundness above my pubic arch—a gesture one part "checking in" and one part protection that had started unconsciously the moment I knew I was pregnant and had since become reflex. I removed my coat and fiddled with my handbag to give my restless hands something else to do. The little pooch in my abdomen barely showed beneath my long, knit shirt; I didn't have to tell anyone I was pregnant if I didn't want to. Uneasiness and uncertainty were the overriding feelings that skulked within. Absent was the joyous expectation that usually accompanies a much-wanted pregnancy. Even hope had vanished, given up after three failed attempts to have a baby. Better to feel as little as possible.

I met my soon-to-be sister-in-law's mother and many of the rest of her female relatives. One sister had traveled from out of town and shared a photo album filled with pictures—mostly of a handsome dog.

I fixed a plate of food and found myself seated next to the grandmother, and immediately feared I'd made a mistake. What if she wanted to grill me about her granddaughter's fiancé—my husband's brother? That was a subject I knew even less about than babies. Oh, I knew all about getting pregnant. But babies? I was scared to death of having one—and even more scared of losing another one. Though I told myself that the miscarriages were no reflection on my mothering abilities, deep down I had doubts. I thought back to the dog pictures. My husband and I had a big, black Lab. Why hadn't I just stuck with a dog—stuck with what I knew?

One of the other women sitting at the table asked, "Now, is your husband the oldest in his family?"

"He's the second, after the twins," I explained, feeling my chest tighten in anticipation of the barrage of questions to follow.

But the third-degree didn't happen. They were pleasant, and I relaxed. If I didn't reveal I was pregnant, no one would be the wiser. There was no reason to hide it, really, except for that pervading uncertainty. Only in the past few days had I felt my baby moving, like a little fish swimming around my belly. Surely no one could blame me for wanting to keep that to myself?

My high-risk pregnancy required extra care. After myriad tests and procedures that required lots of blood work and time with my feet in the stirrups, an astute doctor had finally discovered the reason for my losses—an autoimmune disorder called elevated ANA. A woman's body is supposed to nurture and shelter a fetus; mine had attacked and rejected ours like nasty viruses or unwanted transplants. This pregnancy I gave myself injections of a blood thinner every day to prevent miscarriage. My steadily growing belly wore a chain of blue bruises from the daily needle pricks. The doctor had assured us that everything would be all right. Still, even though I very much wanted to make known my condition, I had an unreasonable fear of telling, as if letting the cat out of the bag might somehow jinx it.

My husband, Robert, shared my concern, perhaps felt it even more strongly, since he couldn't feel the baby, safe inside, like I did. But he didn't show his fear, and I tried to contain mine. When I was pregnant the first time, we told everyone as soon as we knew. The second time we decided to wait a bit longer before saying anything. We had mentioned it only to close family when, at about seven weeks, I awoke one night with severe pain in my abdomen. Robert dialed 911 with one hand and held on to me with the other. I could barely breathe as I listened to him give my symptoms and our address.

"Tell them I'm pregnant," I said between gasps. I thought it might be important.

"Oh," he said. "Right." Then, to the operator, "And we think she might be pregnant."

The next day, after we learned it was a gall bladder attack and had nothing to do with the baby, I asked him what he meant when he said, "And we think she might be pregnant."

"Well," he said, "I wasn't sure who we were telling yet."

Although his caution with the 911 operator

seemed overdone, I laughed. A week later I lost that baby, and the next pregnancy ended at eleven weeks. After losing three babies in three years, I grew angry and swore off charting my morning temperature, tracking my cycle week after week, and taking an ovulation test every month. But then nature took her course. So, there I was, forty-one years old, in my fourth pregnancy, feeling unsure about everything. No matter what the doctor said, I kept hope tamped down and the "good news" to myself. The fewer who knew, the fewer I'd have to call if things didn't work out again.

With several generations of women gathered in one place, the conversation inevitably turned to children as we waited for the bride-to-be to arrive. Of course, these women were naturally curious about her future husband's siblings and their families, and I was the only spokesperson present. I figured I could report what I knew but keep my condition hidden.

"There are five siblings in their family," I said. "His sister also has five children, and his oldest brother has four." Several heads nodded. They had, no doubt, heard this before, but they double-checked names and birth order to be sure.

"The youngest brother has two children," I continued, cringing inwardly as their gazes sharpened.

"What about you and Robert? How long did you say you've been married?"

I had already let it slip that we had been married over eight years, but I hadn't mentioned any children. Clearly, I was not going to get anything past this crowd. Though I had been determined not to mention I was expecting, an urge to speak crept up my throat like a niggling cough, as though my baby was insisting on being known. The women's warmth invited trust. *But what if I lost the baby again?* I wondered. *They would find out soon enough, anyway, it might as well be from me,* I countered. Uneasiness warred with desire. Desire won.

"Well, actually, I'm pregnant," I said … and then added, "Right now," as if it needed clarification.

The grandmother clapped her hands. "That's wonderful!"

The energy in the room swelled like my budding belly. No one moved, yet I felt them shift toward me, as if I were at the center of an embracing and protective inner circle.

"Do you know whether it's a boy or girl?" someone asked.

"We're not sure yet." But I planned to find out. I wanted to know, even though it made no difference as long as the baby was healthy.

"When are you due?"

"August twenty-fourth."

"Oh, I was pregnant in the summer, too. How have you been feeling?"

"Fine. No morning sickness."

"Gawd," another woman said. "I was sick, and not just in the mornings. Couldn't stand the smell of coffee, and I love coffee."

"Do you plan on breastfeeding?" someone asked.

"Oh, yes, for as long as possible."

"I just weaned my youngest, and she's three."

As I answered their questions and they shared their own experiences, my trepidation abated. Then, just when I was feeling relaxed, came the dreaded question.

"Is this your first?"

I hesitated. "This is my fourth pregnancy." I took a deep breath. "I've had three miscarriages."

There it was. I'd said it. Out loud. In a room full of people I barely knew. And oddly enough, revealing this intimate and painful fact of my life to these relative strangers didn't cause me distress. Instead, it felt good to talk about it, and my story, along with my tension, poured out. I felt the love and support of these women—many of them mothers—surround me and my baby, pushing away the uncertainty and allowing the joy to seep in.

Pregnancy and birth and baby stories emerged like birds fluttering from cages. Stories of life. Of new lives—each one precious. Of lost lives—as witnessed by those who had miscarried or knew someone who had.

"Remember how hard your second one kicked?"

"You were as big as a house!"

"I felt like I was in labor for days, but oh, how glorious it felt when they laid her in my arms the first time."

"Can you believe how much he cried?"

"He had colic for a few weeks, but then he slept through the night."

"My first didn't sleep through until she was two."

They reminded each other of what the fathers had said or didn't say, and of how nervous they'd been as new moms, changing diapers, nursing, allergies, the dearth or excess of hair, tiny fingers and toes, and first smiles and on and on. They stopped talking only to me and lost themselves in their stories, weaving their family history in the air around us like a warm blanket. They told tales of babies who came early and ones who came late. They told of babies who came easily and those whose entries into the world were more difficult but nonetheless welcomed.

I listened, and though I was not the guest of honor that day, I received the best gift of all—membership in the secret club of motherhood. And somehow I knew everything would be all right. My baby would be all right.

—Candace Carrabus

Like a Natural Woman

I had heard of underwater births, like I'd heard of couples getting married while skydiving. I just didn't think anyone I knew, especially Jillian, was the type to do it. Jillian was one of my closest friends. Since graduate school, we lived almost parallel lives, experiencing many of the same milestones—starting first jobs, getting married, changing jobs, getting pregnant—within a few months of each other. I thought I knew Jillian well, but a few weeks before my due date she surprised me.

"What's your birthing plan?" she asked.

The question seemed as strange as someone asking me to describe my escape plan from a burning building—one of those things I hadn't thought enough about to devise an actual plan and hoped everything would turn out okay when the time came. And pressed to come up with a plan for delivering my baby on the spot, it sounded a lot like what I supposed my strategy for escaping from a burning building would be: "Get out as fast as possible with as little pain as possible."

"No, seriously," Jillian laughed. "Are you planning a natural birth?"

Then I laughed. Wouldn't any delivery short of birthing the baby out of my ear be natural?

Jillian proceeded to tell me about her birthing plan. Though only a few months pregnant, she had already thought through every detail. She was planning on delivering her baby at a birthing center in a birthing pool with the help of a midwife. She used phrases like, "natural transition to the world" and "control over my own body" and ended with the declaration, "No drugs, no hospitals, no doctors."

At first, I felt like the dim-witted student who proudly told the teacher, "Because we wanted to be free," only to be trumped by the teacher's pet who elaborated that rebellion against the Sugar and Stamp Acts and the lack of American representation in Parliament were the causes for the Revolutionary War.

But when Jillian said something about taking her placenta home, I thought she was absolutely crazy. No epidural? There's nothing natural about screaming bloody murder when you aren't being murdered. No hospital? If something were to go wrong, you need Western medicine, modern technology, and a doctor—someone with a university degree who has spent years studying the body and training as a resident, not someone with a certificate from a weekend class offered at Stella's Wellness Center.

"You can't trust hospitals," Jillian explained, sensing my skepticism. "Like any other big business, all they care about is the bottom line." Jillian told me about some report that revealed doctors are increasingly forcing women to have C-sections unnecessarily so that hospitals can charge more and so that doctors can spend more time playing golf. "Especially if you happen to go into labor on a Wednesday."

Jillian's stereotype of doctors offended me. My father was a doctor, and he played golf only on Fridays. And what I remember, more than him heading out to the driving range, was him jumping up from the dinner table, dropping unopened gifts on Christmas morning, and running out of the movie theater to respond to emergency calls. Unlike Jillian, I had complete faith in doctors. The body is a miracle and a mystery to me, like flying an airplane. I have no idea how that massive hunk of metal gets off the ground, but when the pilot tells me to prepare for landing, I'm not about to question him on whether he's sure the landing gear is aligned properly and all of the flaps are up. It boggles my mind to think that something the size of a bowling ball could come out of a three-inch opening. If a doctor tells me a C-section is the best option for me and my baby, I say, sign me up.

"Not only that," Jillian continued, "hospitals are too cold and clinical. My cousin just delivered at Beth Israel and immediately after the baby came out the nurses whisked it away to do tests or whatever. It was ten whole minutes before she got to see her newborn."

The thought of assuming responsibilities as a mother for the rest of my life was overwhelming and downright scary to me. As far as I was concerned, the nurses could take as much time as needed after the delivery before officially passing me the torch. No, it would take more than that to get me to sign up for a deep-sea delivery.

By the time I relayed Jillian's birthing plan to John that evening, I had reduced it to "squatting over a bucket of water."

"Like she's taking a dump," my husband, John, as appalled as I was, added.

My due date came, but my baby did not. By the time I was two weeks overdue, I had given up hope of experiencing my water breaking in the middle of the night and the excitement of rushing to the hospital. I made an appointment to have my labor induced. On the scheduled date, I cleaned the bathroom, checked e-mails, and enjoyed a leisurely dinner with John before heading to the hospital.

"I'm here to deliver my baby," I chirped to the receptionist in the prenatal wing. A women in labor who was trudging down the hall hunched over like a ninety-year-old man glared at me. *How dare you be so happy,* her eyes read. As soon as I settled into the hospital bed, a nurse inserted a tablet into my cervix.

"That oughtta jump-start things," she said.

She wasn't lying. Within the hour my contractions started. I felt mild cramps, like I had eaten too much spicy shrimp pad thai, but I called for the anesthesiologist before it got any worse. He came immediately with his long, extremely intimidating needle.

"Make it a double," I joked.

He must have taken me seriously, because after the sting of the needle in my back faded, I couldn't feel a thing from my waist down. My contractions progressed quickly, or so the nurses told me. I was oblivious to what my body was doing as I watched back-to-back episodes of *Law & Order.* Just as the rapist was about to break down and confess everything, Dr. Berger came in and put my feet up on the stirrups. John took out the camcorder.

This is it, I thought. *The moment I have been waiting nine months for is finally here. I'm going to bring a human being into this world. I'm going to become a mother.*

"Is that a Sony Digital8?" Dr. Berger asked. For the next twenty minutes, John and my obstetrician clamored on about pixel count, LCD display panels, and optical zoom range.

"Okay, now push," Dr. Berger ordered, bringing attention back to the real reason why we were all gathered around my vagina. "Excellent, now again. Good, good. The head is almost out."

Unbelievable. Only two pushes and I was nearly done? I pushed like I was constipated, but by no means was I exerting myself. I felt like I was cheating, getting off too easy. My delivery would never be aired on the Discovery Health Channel.

I decided to fake a little pain to give the appearance that bringing life into the world was taking some effort. The next time Dr. Berger ordered me to push, I added a few grunts. On subsequent pushes, I gritted my teeth for further effect. Then I really got into it and let out a big moan for the grand finale, "Auuugh!"

John, Dr. Berger, and the nurses looked up at me like I was the only one left singing in church after the rest of congregation ended. The baby had already come out.

The nurses whisked away my baby to a far corner in the room, just as Jillian had warned. I thought it was mighty polite of them, however, to wash off the slimy, bloody alien that came from my body before handing me a clean, adorable baby wrapped snugly, like a burrito, in a blanket. Everything was perfect. Things couldn't have gone better had I planned it.

Jillian gave birth several months later. She called to tell me she was having contractions and was on her way to the birthing center.

"Good luck," I told her, secretly hoping the baby's huge head would get stuck as she squatted over her bucket, causing so much pain she'd beg to be taken to the hospital for an epidural. Jillian called the next morning. Everything went according to plan. The experience was beautiful, and she did it without drugs, without a hospital, and without doctors. Judgment oozed from the phone like jelly out of a squished donut.

There were so many times I wanted to confide in Jillian—new mother to new mother—how frustrated I felt when Gregory squirmed when I tried to change him or how desperately I wanted to smear the poopy diaper in John's face when he stood over me, directing me to wipe there and there and not to forget that spot there. But I feared our conversation would end with me writing down a number for her cloth diaper delivery service and feeling even worse.

Jillian and I drifted apart. We stopped calling each other, and eventually our only communication was the occasional e-mail apologizing for not calling, blaming it on our busy lives as working mothers. But the truth is, we avoided each other because I'm sure as much as I was thinking, *Give me a break. You're taking this motherhood thing way too seriously,* when Jillian told me about how Olivia just loves the mashed organic carrots and squash recipe she makes from her Gourmet Baby cookbook, she was thinking, *Are you kidding? You're not serious enough to be a mother,* when I proudly reported that Gregory watches the entire Baby Einstein video—all 45 minutes of it.

There were many times when I wondered whether I was wrong and Jillian was right. Maybe Gregory was so colicky at night because he hadn't had a natural transition to the world by being born underwater. Then there was the two-week period when I was convinced Gregory hated me. He screamed whenever I came near him and would let only his father pick him up. I wondered whether my son would ever bond with me, given the fact that I wasn't there for him during the first ten minutes of his life. Things gradually improved, however. Gregory started sleeping through the night, and there was a two-week stretch when he loved me again and hated John.

Feeling more confident in my abilities as a mother, I decided to give Jillian a call one evening. I missed her. And I was curious to know whether or not she was still making organic baby food from scratch, using cloth diapers, and enforcing a no-TV policy. Jillian answered, and I could hear Olivia screaming in the background.

"Can I call you back?" a frazzled-sounding Jillian asked.

I was disappointed we didn't get a chance to talk, but I was also relieved to know her baby cries too, despite being born underwater. I hung up the phone and turned on the TV. I had tried to read Gregory his bedtime story before calling Jillian, but he'd protested, "I wan Dada!" No problem. I welcomed the opportunity to watch *Law & Order*, knowing that phase would pass all too soon.

—*Elizabeth Ridley*

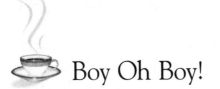# Boy Oh Boy!

I've always dreamed of having a little girl of my own. It wasn't that I was a girlie girl or that I was particularly fond of little kids. I never played with dolls, preferring to wrestle with my younger brother or to run around outside with the neighborhood kids. As an adolescent, I didn't care much for babysitting, unless I needed to earn pocket change to pay for my next Bon Jovi or Duran Duran album. Still, I always knew I would have a daughter someday.

I also decided early on that I would name her Katherine, after my mother and grandmother, both of whom insisted on being called Kate. My parents had almost named me Katherine, too, but then decided at the last minute to make Katherine my middle name to avoid confusion. Kate is a strong, confident, feminine name—the characteristics my daughter would surely possess. She would be like the other Kates—intelligent, creative women who followed their passions.

The original Kate, my grandmother, paid her way through the University of Chicago and met Pop while in the university's graduate program. Raising their three daughters and two sons kept her housebound but not constrained. She would often drop the laundry basket or dash from the kitchen to grab the typewriter she kept on the sofa, resting it on her knees to capture a thought that she would eventually polish into a perceptive essay. Most of her many published works focus on the issues of women and motherhood.

Her oldest child, my mother, the second Kate, followed her own dreams in the theater and became a well-known local actress. Later, she parlayed her skills into her own executive training business. She continues to teach me, her own oldest child, how to live an authentic and fulfilling life.

I've often thought about my future daughter— what I would teach her, how I would raise her, and what she would be inspired to do for herself. I would encourage her to follow her own interests in school, whether ballet or football. I would teach her to respect herself and her body, and never to lose sight of who she was. As a young woman, she would travel the world, stand up for the rights of all women, and be an active contributor to society.

When I became pregnant with my first child, I didn't need an ultrasound to tell me it was a girl. I was completely in tune with my body and my baby. I practiced yoga and meditated daily, and at night I dreamed of the little girl growing inside of me. When the midwife handed me my new baby boy, I looked into his big blue eyes and was as happy as could be. Besides, the next one would be a girl.

Exactly two years later, I was in the delivery room, anxious to meet my daughter. This time, when my husband said, "It's another boy!" I had a moment of shock, of disbelief, of near panic. Where was my girl—the girl to whom I'd teach everything I had learned, the girl who wouldn't make the mistakes I had made, the girl who would become an independent, confident woman? I even wondered who would keep me well-groomed and dignified when I grew old, too old to manage the tweezers.

Those concerns, of course, subsided when I was handed my second son. He was perfect. As he began to nurse, I was overcome with love for him and guilt for expecting someone else.

Now, my boys, ages two and four, keep my days filled with dirty diapers, muddy pants, cuts and bruises, tears, and drippy noses, followed by nights disturbed by kicks from a child who has made his way from his bed to ours. Despite the chaos, every day brings me joy, usually in small, seemingly insignificant ways. Maybe it is my two-year-old surprising me with a well-spoken full sentence. Or my four-year-old making me laugh when he asks if he can someday go to the top of the "Serious Tower."

On this particular day, my boys are side by side on the floor, concentrating on their LEGO projects. I am enlightened by the rare moment of peace, free from the noise and energy of boyish rowdiness. I sit on the couch observing them, grateful that I do not have to play referee or nurse or teacher.

Jack, my oldest, looks at his brother and asks, "Could I have your yellow block, Will?"

Will hesitates for a second and then hands the block to his brother.

Instead of saying "thank you," Jack says matter-of-factly, "I love you, Will."

Will, without looking up from his blocks or removing his pacifier, dutifully replies, "I love you, too."

At that moment, I realized that I might never have the daughter I had always envisioned, but it didn't mean I would not have children with the attributes of my imagined Kate. Instead, I have been blessed with two kind, generous, and sensitive boys. As their mother, I can foster their natural tenderness and their respect for each other, for women, for all people. They will grow into sensitive men who will recognize the struggles too often experienced by women that I thought only daughters could fully recognize. They will become men who are in touch with their emotions and who know how to act on those feelings to make things better. Compassion, strength of character, and individuality are integral parts of my sons' lineage—in the tradition of the two great Kates. That, I also realized, is an incredibly precious and all-too-rare gift to the world.

—*Anne O'Connor Bodine*

Tea Parties Aren't Mandatory

Everything changed the day I refused to go into the bathroom. You see, I've never been altogether comfortable with my role as a female in this world. Raised as an only child by a single father, I got my kicks on the back of my dad's motorcycle and under the hood of a car rather than at tea parties and sleepovers. Oh, I cleaned up well enough. Dad bought me pretty dresses to wear to church and even learned how to operate a curling iron . . . sort of.

"Did you plug it in?"

"Yes, I plugged it in."

"Did you turn it on?"

"Yes, Rachel, I turned it on."

"Well, what are we waiting for?"

"The dot is supposed to turn red."

"What dot?"

"That one," he said pointing at the little black spot on top of the chrome clasp.

"It looks hot to me."

"Let me see," he said as he snatched it away. "Ouch!"

"I told you it was hot."

"Just read the directions."

"Where did they go? Oh, here they are." I quickly scanned the directions. "Dad, it doesn't turn red. It starts out red and turns black."

"All right, all right. Now what do we do?"

So it continued at every feminine turn in my development. When it came time for me to wear a bra, my teacher sent home a note that made my father blush.

"'Mr. Gibson,'" he read aloud. "'Rachel is at the point in her development that requires her to wear a—' . . . Oh. . . . Um. . . . Okay."

He handed over the note, his JCPenney credit card, and me to the saleslady while he stood outside the department of "unmentionables" with his shoes butted against the edge of the red carpet as if it were smoldering lava that might consume him with his next step.

"Come on, Dad."

"No, that's okay. I'm sure you can handle it from here."

When I was a little girl, I would sit on the edge of the tub while my dad, clad only in his briefs, would sing, "Hey Good Lookin'" to his reflection while shaving. After my period started, I never saw him in his underwear again nor were we ever in the bathroom at the same time again.

Every step of my journey toward womanhood passed the same way—tainted by an eerie sense of discomfort and guilt. And I felt everything was my fault . . . for being a girl.

Of course, as I got older, my unconventional upbringing sometimes worked in my favor. Because my father always treated me like "one of the boys," I became a force to be reckoned with. I had a competitive edge that many girls lack. I competed with women and won. I competed with men and won. I finished college near the top of my class and had a string of successful jobs before striking out on my own as an independent rock band promoter—a highly competitive field dominated by men.

I loved my life, but being one of the guys had its disadvantages too. For one thing, aside from professional and platonic relationships, men wouldn't come near me. When it came to romance, I was unapproachable, maybe even a little scary. But Jon changed all of that.

Unlike the stereotypical rock 'n roll drummer, Jon was a quiet, soft-spoken sweetheart. Unlike other men, he treated me as an equal but also as a woman, and he wasn't intimidated by me or my career. He became my best friend, and then the love of my life, and eventually my husband. Best of all, he didn't find me scary or unapproachable in the least. For the first time in my life, someone really saw "me"—all of me.

"Tomboy" no longer applied. Some baggage, though, never goes away, and I was still a selfish only child. So, I turned what most people seemed to think was a fatal flaw into my badge of honor, adopting the mantra: "I'm too selfish to have children." Family and friends accepted my declaration of selfishness without too much ado, figuring, I suppose, that at least I'd been self-aware and honest enough to admit it.

Then, everything changed the day I refused to go into the bathroom. I'd managed to wade through the muck of denial and dread enough to acknowledge that I needed to take the test and then to drag myself to the store to buy it. I'd even managed, with a detached steadiness, to read and follow the directions. But that was as far as I could go.

"Time's up," I muttered.

"Let's go have a look."

"I'm not looking."

"Rachel, you're acting like a child."

"Maybe. But I'm not going, and you can't make me."

"Rachel, the results will be the same whether you go in with me or I go in alone."

"Fine. It's settled. You go in."

"All right. Be that way."

No words were necessary when Jon exited the bathroom. I could tell by the how-am-I-going-to-get-her-through-this look on his face. My world started to crumble.

"I cannot be pregnant. I won't."

"You won't? How old are you? You can't refuse to be pregnant."

"I'm too selfish to have kids."

"That may be true, but that doesn't make you any less pregnant."

"What about my job?"

"What about your job? You're self-employed. Who's going to fire you?"

"I'm a rock band promoter."

"I remember. Rock stars have mothers too," he said with a smile.

"Funny. I'm sure I'm going to look just fabulous in leather pants when I'm nine months pregnant."

"Well, at least you're not refusing to be pregnant anymore. That's progress."

"What about our apartment?" I asked.

"The baby isn't going to fit."

"I'm not moving."

"Rachel, what are we going to do, put the baby under the bed?"

"See? The baby isn't even here, and already everything's changing. I'm going to have to share my time, my space, you."

"Yes, and we'll—"

"Oh no!"

"What?"

"What if I have a girl?"

"Oh no!" he mocked me. "Look," he tried to reason, "you're a girl, and that's worked out all right."

"I am not a girl."

"A woman, then."

"I am not a woman."

"We are running out of options," he laughed.

"I'm not kidding. I'm really not a girl."

"Honey, you're fine. You'll be beautiful—leather pants and all. We'll probably have a boy, anyway. And if you don't, remember, tea parties aren't mandatory. We'll deal with the rest as it comes."

He was right, as usual. I was beautiful in leather pants, if I do say so myself, and we did have a boy—our little Oscar. He's the second love of my life. He's the joy in my days; I can't imagine my life without him in it. Now, finally, I am comfortable with being a girl, a woman, a wife, and a mother—my way. Because, after all, tea parties aren't mandatory.

—*R. L. Gibson*

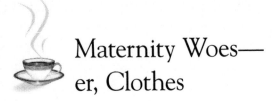

Maternity Woes— er, Clothes

For months, I had eagerly awaited the arrival of a certain bundle of joy . . . my first bag of maternity hand-me-downs.

Shortly after I announced the impending birth of my first child, boxes and bags filled with used maternity clothing were bestowed upon me along with the well wishes. At first I was baffled and mildly insulted. What fashion faux pas had I unknowingly committed that made other women feel compelled to clothe me with their closet discards? With pregnancy, had I suddenly lost the capacity to shop along with my ability to take out the trash without gagging and to go more than forty minutes without a bathroom break? Under normal, nongestational circumstances, we well-attired women would never think of wearing cast-offs from friends, family, and neighbors, much less friends of friends, family, and neighbors, and certainly not from casual acquaintances and total strangers. We would never consider asking for old outfits to use for six months or more, after which we would return them so they could be passed on to countless others. But after a brief tour through the strange and frightening dimension of maternity shopping, this practice suddenly seemed perfectly acceptable.

My first stop at a local department store was quite enlightening. Way in the back of the store, under a flickering fluorescent light and a leaky ceiling, was The Maternity Dungeon, er, Department. It consisted of two racks of the least attractive clothing I had ever seen. The odd assortment of apparel also looked as though it had been designed when Ralph Lauren's great grandparents were in vitro. It smelled that way, too. So I quickly moved on.

The mall had a clothing store dedicated to expectant mothers. *Eureka!* I thought. *Surely, I'll have better luck here.* Indeed, the selection was much improved; some of the stuff was even attractive, comfortable, and contemporary, or at least one of those. This handy-dandy maternity boutique offered items dedicated to parts of my body I didn't know I had before. They even provided pillows of various sizes in the dressing rooms to propel yourself to five months, six months, seven months, eight months, and nine months along—as if to suggest that the only place in which there would be any weight gain was in that cute little tummy. Looking back, perhaps pillows dedicated to the arms, thighs, chest, and buttocks might have been equally beneficial.

I tried on the selections with relish, quickly loading my cart with a variety of treasures. However, upon reaching the cash register, I discovered that not only was I now eating for two, I also was paying for seven. Apparently, dressing like a semi-normal person during pregnancy comes with a stiff price. That elastic pouch in the front of a pair of jeans must cost manufacturers a bundle to install, because that is the only difference I could see that might explain the substantially higher price. And that little bit of extra fabric added to T-shirts, blouses, sweaters, and dresses to cover swollen bellies must go for $100 a yard and be hand-woven with the finest fibers to warrant those price tags.

So I had a few choices: Blow my entire wardrobe budget for the next five years on clothing I would wear for five months. Blow my entire budget for the baby's nursery and layette, and let the kid go naked and sleep in a drawer for six months. Or put some . . . okay, most . . . of the stuff back.

Suddenly, all of those offers of used, free clothing didn't sound quite so distasteful. But still . . . a clothes horse doesn't go down easily.

I tried the only other two maternity shops in the county, putting a few hundred miles on my car and on my aching back with the same discouraging results. Maternity shopping was not child's play. Then reluctantly, I made the call to my sister-in-law. The surrender of my fashion dignity was brief, and the ceremony was scheduled.

Unbeknownst to me, I was about to embark upon an ancient maternal ritual passed through generations like some sort of feminine bonding rite. My sister-in-law bequeathed to me the Holy Grail of Maternity Wear: a bag filled with skirts from A Pea in the Pod, waistless dresses, and oversized overalls. It was like I had hit the mother lode! I grabbed the bag greedily, but she admonished me quickly.

She told me in no uncertain terms that this was merely a rental, a month-to-month tenancy not to exceed, oh, nine or so months. There would be nothing sisterly about the behavior that resulted if I were to upset the chain by holding on to the communal wraps beyond my lease or, heaven forbid, by lending them to an unauthorized person. Generations would be destroyed if that bag detoured from its predestined lineage.

I nodded my assent as I spied a pair of support hose peeking out. A shiver of dread ran up my spine.

It wasn't quite as bad as I thought it would be. Not quite. During those first weeks while the novelty was still firmly in place, I was almost giddy about my blossoming-with-child body and my new used-wardrobe. I thought my slightly rotund tummy and slight waddle were cute. I could still see my toes, my ankle bones were still visible, and my backside was still an appropriate girth. I humbly wore the nicest (and smallest) hand-me-downs and stuffed the rest back into the bag, laughing at the absurdity of their size.

As the months wore on, the clothing got tighter. The elastic cut into places on my body I could no longer reach. During those last waning weeks, I surfed the Internet for a Ringling Bros. catalog, thinking a circus tent might soon be my only option. I thought about requesting that my baby shower be a toga party, so I would at least have something comfortable to wear. Even the clothing labels were cutting into my bloated flesh, and those larger items I had so cavalierly exiled to the bottom of the bag were now stretched to capacity over stretch marks.

I couldn't wait for the baby's due date, not only for his joyous arrival but also so I could abandon my secondhand trousseau. For some absurd reason, I had it in my mind that I would walk out of the delivery ward carrying my new son and wearing a size 6 pair of jeans and a halter top. Oh, how wrong I was. Apparently, a few days and four sit-ups were not going to bring me anywhere near my closet. Though my fashion sense returned postpartum, my waist did not. Neither did my chest, backside, or thighs. I resigned myself to my hand-me-downs for an undetermined length of time, hoping I could bid them good riddance before my child was old enough to be embarrassed by his mother's appearance.

Months later, I met my sister-in-law at the mall with the complete contents of that original bundle of almost a year prior. She was thankful, saying that her cousin's foster mother's brother's daughter was eagerly awaiting the garments. I smiled with a newfound appreciation. As we headed toward a store where I hoped to pick out a few items to fit my slowly returning frame, we passed an expectant mother. A rosy tint highlighted her cheeks.

"Ah, she's glowing," my sister-in-law said.

But I knew better. That flushed face had little to do with hormones. More so, it came from the frustration and humiliation of having just realized that finding affordable, attractive maternity clothes was about as likely as winning the lottery . . . and that she would soon be wearing who-knows-what kind of hand-me-downs from who-knows-where.

—*Tracey Henry*

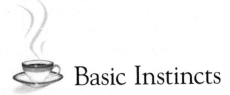 Basic Instincts

I saved my baby's life before she was even born.

Of course, any parent can lay claim to a life saved. What mother hasn't performed the Heimlich maneuver on an infant choking on his sister's Barbie shoe, retrieved a toddler who's slipped under four inches of bath water, or rescued a child from any of the thousand dangers they find so irresistible? Human babies are born without the capacity to defend themselves, and many of us take on the role of bodyguard with the ferocity of mercenary soldiers. But even as an experienced mommy, it's not always easy to follow your gut when medical professionals are telling you otherwise.

When I was pregnant with my second child, I was obsessively worried about my impending delivery. My first child was two steamy July weeks overdue, and after a macabre induction resulting in a cesarean birth, I was twice as anxious the second time around. I wanted so badly to deliver naturally, to prove to myself that I could endure the most physical of trials. I thought that perhaps I would feel more like a "real" mother if I could control my birthing experience. My doctor told me to relax and said I would probably go into labor if I stopped fretting so much.

A few days before the baby was due, I took my husband to his office, about thirty minutes away. My back began to ache on the way home, and I chalked it up to our ancient Honda's unyielding bucket seats. I tried napping, but I couldn't find a position comfortable enough for my swollen body. Instead of the regular, rhythmic contractions I had read about, I was experiencing constant pain, and my temperature was rising, though I felt very cold.

My mother and my husband fed me take-out wonton soup and eventually drove me to the hospital. I remember thinking that this pregnancy business was a very bad idea, and if I could get to the ER in one piece, maybe I could make a deal with the doctors that if they would sort it all out, I would never so much as consider having another baby again—if I could just dodge delivering this one now.

I was examined and re-examined, my temperature taken and my uterus awkwardly prodded by a succession of embarrassingly handsome residents. The verdict? We don't know.

The medical professionals agreed that I was in labor and slowly dilating, and that an infection somewhere in my body was probably spiking my fever. What they couldn't figure out was whether it was my baby or me or both of us who had the infection. Their recommendation was to get a good night's rest at the hospital and begin an induction first thing in the morning. I gratefully accepted a sedative, but awoke hourly to pee. Every hour on the hour my mother got out of the crackly vinyl chair at the foot of my bed and helped me navigate my IV and monitor cords to and from the bathroom, and then tucked me tenderly back into bed and talked quietly about unimportant things until I went back to sleep.

In the morning, the resident gave me the induction hard-sell. I was so afraid to relive the "failed induction" of my first birth, and hoped that it was me and not the baby who was sick. Why didn't they know what was wrong? As much as I wanted a natural childbirth, as much as I feared another cesarean, I made a decision.

"I think we had better get her out now. Give me the C-section, and we'll figure it all out when she's safe."

The doctors didn't love this idea; they were uncomfortable with such a drastic escalation. My husband, groggy from a night of sleeping on a plastic recliner, reminded me of our birth plan and my wish for a nonsurgical birth. It was a brave speech. But my mother reared up and shouted, "It's her body, and she can have a C-section if she wants!" He hastily agreed. Unfortunately, the doctors kept trying to convince me otherwise, reminding me that a cesarean is major surgery and, like marriage, not to be entered into lightly. Stubbornly, I insisted—and prevailed.

The actual surgery is a montage, not a narrative, in my memory. I recall my husband almost passing out when he left his station by my head to see our newborn daughter, Alice, lifted out of me. I remember the efficient, hollow silence of the delivery room that meant things had gone wrong, and feeling panicky and helpless when they determined she wasn't getting enough oxygen and rushed her to neonatal intensive care. She was there for eight hours or so, tubes in her nose, and it seemed like years passed before anyone remembered me, marooned in my hospital bed, too worried to do anything but stare. I was glad my husband was with our daughter, so she wouldn't be alone as well. I tried to get out of bed to find her, but I couldn't move my body. I have never felt so helpless, so powerless, in my whole life.

Afterward, my husband told me how they slid my daughter out of my abdomen and asked him to call out the sex and cut the cord. How lightheaded he felt when he saw the surgeon unwrap the umbilical cord from our baby's purple neck, once, twice, three times. And how the doctors in the room remarked that they had never seen anything like it. Later, we learned that she would not have tolerated induction or labor, because the entire length of the cord was wound around her neck, and trying to push her out might have strangled her. Had I followed the doctors' recommendations and attempted a natural delivery, an emergency C-section would have been the most optimistic outcome. My decision—the "elective cesarean," for which they billed us—made it possible for my daughter to receive the care that saved her life. My own general practitioner said, "I will never doubt your intuition again."

Exuberant family and friends filled our tiny hospital room. We went home, moved on, grew up some more, and that blue baby girl is an active, beautiful four-year-old who loves to dance and thinks the world is full of friends she hasn't yet met.

Ever since, whenever I'm tempted to doubt my "mother's intuition," to listen to someone's advice instead of my own inner voice, I remember the fear and pride I felt that day, challenging a roomful of physicians and nurses, standing strong despite my fear. I'm grateful for the hospital staff's quick, skilled intervention after my daughter was born, but I wish they had listened to me sooner. Nobody knows my body or my babies better than I do, and no one can make decisions for my children better than I can.

This one instant in my life—the tiny second when time slowed and my pulse drummed in my head and I heard my own voice in my heart—is the moment I hold tightly when I worry about my children now.

Every woman wonders whether she has what it takes to be a mom. We all know that motherhood is in the "doing"—in the endless care and feeding and physical attendance—but it's also in the "being," in those long months of growing a baby cell by cell and in knowing that you are ultimately responsible for that life. I have a connection with my daughter that is eternal and unparalleled, at least until she has a child of her own. And in between the rock and the hard place, between life and death, there is a quiet space inside me where I know I have the power to do anything necessary to keep my children safe. Mothers know these things.

—*Gwyn Rhoades*

The Master Plan

I'd pinpointed my date of ovulation and conceived on schedule, planning the birth of my future baby so that it wouldn't interfere with vacations or holidays. Aside from some morning sickness, everything had progressed according to my plan.

Or so I'd thought.

Sixteen weeks into my pregnancy, I found myself bloated with quarts of water, wearing nothing but panties and a flimsy gown and lying in a darkened cubicle. The ultrasound technician, a young woman named Angie, squeezed a coil of clear jelly onto my bare abdomen. The instant the cold lubricant hit my skin, I shivered and my distended bladder responded by threatening to let loose. Crossing my ankles tightly, I contracted my pelvic muscles to resist the urge to urinate. Angie stuck the wand in the goo and rolled it over my belly like she was applying a coat of varnish.

To add to my discomfort, the aroma of coffee steaming in her mug nauseated me. Holding my breath, I turned my head to stifle a gag and noticed a poster tacked to the wall depicting fetal development. While I willed my stomach to settle, I stared at it, pretending I was comfortable lying half-naked on a hard table while a stranger plumbed my reproductive organs with a device developed for submarine warfare.

Abruptly, the wand stopped below my navel, stayed there for a few chilling seconds, circled and came back around to the same spot, and then hovered there like a predatory bird honing in on its prey. Alarmed, I watched as Angie squinted at the screen and made minute adjustments to the wand's position. Finally, she peered over the monitor, the bluish-silver light from the screen illuminating her face.

"The doctor was right," she said flatly, her face expressionless as she searched mine for a reaction. "See." She swung the monitor around.

Stunned by her words, I looked at the screen. My heart pounded in my chest, blood rushed to my head, and tears filled my eyes, blurring my vision. The picture on the screen swam before me.

Angie turned the monitor back. "Let me take a few pictures, and then I'll get your husband."

I nodded and closed my eyes as tears slid from the corners, rolled down the sides of my face, and spilled into my ears. I dabbed at them, struggling to keep from falling apart, while the technician snapped picture after picture as if I were some newly discovered planet and she was in charge of supplying NASA with photos.

When Angie escorted my husband into the room, he looked at me, his brows arched in question. I nodded my head and mouthed a "yes." He searched my face for a reaction, but I gave none. I couldn't. I didn't want to lose it completely in front of Angie. This was too private a moment to share with a stranger.

My husband pulled up a stool and sat next to me. His cold hand took my clammy, trembling one. The technician swung the monitor back so that it faced both of us. "See," she said in the same flat tone.

My husband gripped my fingers as we gazed into my womb. I struggled to make sense of the view, but then like one of those black and white pictures that can been seen either as a witch or a beautiful girl, my vision sharpened and the image on the screen suddenly became clear.

What a fool I'd been. I'd planned everything, every last detail. But as I peered into my own uterus, it was clear that a party was going on—and I hadn't been invited. Two tadpole babies jumped in my womb, bouncing off its walls like lunatics in a padded cell. Their dark, hollow, fetal eyes and wide-open mouths made them look like smiley-face buttons sprung to life. Hands waved back and forth as they leaped in an exuberant dance of life.

Twins. I definitely had not planned this.

How could this happen in my own body without my knowing it? Clearly, I wasn't as in control as I had thought, if I'd ever had any control at all. I felt like a parent coming home to discover her teenagers throwing a house party. I wanted to grab my belly, shake it, and call into them, "Knock it off in there. And who gave you permission to throw a party?"

As I continued to watch in amazement, I wondered whether the monitor was a window into my future. I saw those babies, my party animal babies, carrying on, and I saw all the other parties yet to come: double baptisms, double birthdays, double proms, double graduations—double trouble. Fate had taken the pieces of my well-ordered, well-planned life and tossed them like confetti into the wind.

"You're done," Angie said as she shut off the monitor. "Congratulations."

As she wiped the jelly from my stomach, my husband patted my shoulder, a saggy smile spread between the corners of his mouth. His pathetic expression caused my eyes to fill up again. As soon as my abdomen was clean, I hopped from the table and ran to the restroom outside the cubicle. He chased after me, but the bathroom door closed behind me, clipping his words. Dashing into a stall, I sat on the toilet, peeing and crying.

After I settled down, I washed my hands, wiped my face, and opened the door. My husband was still standing on the other side, his face pale.

"You didn't want twins, did you?" he asked quietly.

A sob racked my chest and ruffled my lower lip.

Disappointed, he slumped against the wall, looking like he'd acquired my morning sickness.

I picked up the hem of my hospital gown and wiped my eyes. "Oh, I've never been happier," I sniffled. "Did you see them?" I asked, touching his arm. "Our babies—they waved at us."

My husband straightened up, and the color came back into his face. "But the way you ran out of here . . . I thought you didn't—"

I threw my arms around him, hugged him, and said, "I just had to pee so badly. I want twins. I've always wanted twins. I just didn't know it until now."

He squeezed me tightly. Closing my eyes, I watched the shower of colors the confetti of my life made as it fluttered and floated in the air and then settled into a mosaic—a mosaic so magnificent my limited, little mind could have never planned it for me. In that moment I realized there truly is a Master Planner at work who knows our heart's desire even before we do. I thanked Him for not allowing my narrow, foolish plans to crowd out His beautiful, glorious, grander one.

—Janice Lane Palko

Birth of a Nathan

The baby shocked me out of myself. Lying in the bed with the nurse, Patty, who I had met hours before, now seated between my legs on a spinny stool, cheering me on like the coach sister I never had, and all these months of waiting and harboring the seven-pound ball of baby, and then he snakes out of me silent, like a breath of frozen air, and there he is, blue, wrapped in the cord loosely, and the newly appeared on-call doctor that I've never met holds up the baby and then hands him over to me, flops him on my stomach, and I can't remember this part, this seeing the baby. The nurses are scurrying around rattling things, like a bunch of 1840s church women clanking pots and pans and dishes as they prepare for a big church social, and the dad, Barry, my husband, is on my right, and he's breathless and confused, and there's this baby, this wonder mint, this tiny dot of skin, of stillness, of wonder, a blank silent cupcake of love on my left, and I can't catch my breath or my head or my heart, they're all gone. And there are no words for this part—you think there might be words, or at least an image or a special noise or color for this monumental event but there's nothing but this brand new being, a tiny little boy. And wasn't there supposed to be a girl? But here he is, and gone am I, and there is only love.

He is always in motion, arms going in circles, legs going in circles. Impossible to believe I grew that in my stomach, that something so perfect came from someone like me. There must be a God, because I would've forgotten something important. The bridge of the nose. I might've skimped on that. It would've been a drawbridge.

They take the baby to warm him up, and they roll me and my dead legs onto another bed to take me to a room. It's all surreal, because I just spent nine tedious months waiting for the wonder of my life and then in ten minutes he's born, he just slips right out like he's been waiting in line at a buffet and he's just paid, and then people are using his name, Nathan, and now I'm wondering, "Is that a good name?" They're weighing him and footprinting him, and his screams sound like carnival music, and then they wheel me to the other room and I'm put in a bed and given mesh underwear, and my stomach feels like a bean bag, gentle and soft, and I keep putting my hands on it in wonder and kneading it, feeling it pliable, and loving it, my body, the transformation of my body.

Everything's going to my breasts—words, milk, food, family, love, humor, angst—all of it turns into milky liquid, and the baby eats. I have no free hands, nothing frivolous to do with my hands like before, no time for wiping my eyes or a leisurely scratch of the nose. The baby brings loss right to my fingertips, insists he has not taken all my time; he has freed my time. He celebrates my body. He uses me. He cries. He knows exactly what he wants, and it is me, he's sure of it.

The hospital is safe. It's always night, because I'm always in my pajamas and the shades are drawn, and nothing bad ever happens. People come in to tell me various things about my boobs, my bottom half. My family comes in and out, and I can only tell because I hear my mom's high, lilting laugh and I am stapled in with its safety. Nathan and I live like bats in the ceiling of a church—hanging upside down, filled with blood and catching all the faith floating up from below on music.

The nurses surge over us in gentle six-hour waves: "Here's medicine." "Here's food." "Are you all right?" "Isn't he beautiful?" The sunlight comes and goes, and Nathan stays, Nathan's here now. I write his name on a million forms, and I like the shape of his letters, the repetition of the sounds, the way he begins and ends the same way.

It's 3:00 A.M., and he lies in the plastic hospital bassinet beside my hard, narrow, mechanized hospital bed. He's a tiny white mouse, and I feed him all the time, and the light from the bathroom yellows the room into a brown duskiness, and I change my pads and wear the netted underwear and stare at my son, and I can't believe the swirling of the earth around my head.

It is still night, and Barry and I stare at the baby we made, sleeping, no bigger than a pile of spent birthday candles. We look at him because there's nothing else we can do, we're helpless, we're trapped in his sonar, his love grip, and we stare at his little breathing form and sort of glance at each other sideways because it's so packed with emotion it's hard to make eye contact without exploding or disintegrating, and we can't believe we're here, still in the infancy of us and here we are with this brand new life in a hospital room in steamy hot August in Florida.

I get scared of being a mom, of not being able to do it, and Barry tells me, at 3:00 A.M., in his quiet way, "You just have a new friend, that's all," and then he smiles at me.

With this birth I see that everything Barry's been telling me for years is true—that you do everything from your heart. Your brain makes a lot of noise and tries to run things, but you put everything on a shelf and do it from your heart, and you wait and you get things like the birth of a Nathan. Even though everything outside of the little pale plastic hospital bassinet holding Nathan is falling apart, there is hope in this room. Barry keeps coming in and out of my vision, and I can't understand how we've made it this far, and I can't look too closely at the enormity of it all. Like the Grand Canyon. You can focus on only the first hundred feet, the rest is a painting.

—*Juliet Johnson Opper*

"Birth of a Nathan" was first published in *Los Angeles Family Magazine*, August, 2004.

All I Want for Christmas

Outside the frosted panes of our living room window, soft powder puffs of snow fell gently in the hushed expectancy of Christmas Eve. My husband, Ben, and I had just completed the time-honored ritual of hanging stockings and dispensing an assortment of homemade cookies and a glass of milk for Santa Claus. I had tucked our three children into bed amidst a flurry of excitement and last-minute admonitions about what I considered the proper time to rise, even on Christmas morning.

Ben was adjusting a string of Christmas tree lights when I returned to the living room.

"It's the most beautiful tree we've ever had," I told him.

"You say that every year," Ben said with a grin.

He switched on the lights. The tree glowed, bathing the walls in soft gold and amber light. This was the part of Christmas Eve I loved best—Ben and me sitting quietly awaiting the magical hour when we could retrieve the toys and boxes from their secret hideaways and place them lovingly beneath the tree.

As I sank down in the most comfortable chair, a jabbing ache started in my back and worked its way around to my tummy. This was not the first pain; I had been ignoring the telltale signs for almost two hours. My fourth baby had been scheduled to make an appearance on or about the fifteenth of December. I had planned to be home from the hospital before Christmas. December fifteenth had come and gone, but I hadn't. And here it was, Christmas Eve, and I was two weeks overdue and experiencing labor pains.

Maybe it's just another false alarm, I thought, like the time I made the trip to the hospital when I was pregnant with Kathy and had to return home and wait another week.

During the next three hours, the pains came more frequently.

"I think you'd better warm up the car," I broke the news to Ben gently. "I'll phone Mary Catherine to come over." My next-door neighbor had promised to stay with the children when the time came.

"You can't leave now!" Ben looked stricken.

All the days of waiting suddenly came over me. The tears spilled before I could stop them.

"Who will cook the turkey?" I whispered. "I so

wanted to see the children's faces when they opened their gifts under the tree.

"Things will turn out fine," Ben said. He put his arm around me and squeezed me hard. "Don't worry about turkeys or gifts or anything except delivering our new baby into the world. Who knows? Maybe we'll have a Christmas baby."

"A Christmas baby," I repeated slowly. The thought had never occurred to me until then. I dried my eyes. There would be other Christmas mornings to spend with my family.

Ben picked up the overnight bag I had packed two weeks earlier and went outside to start the car. I couldn't resist tiptoeing into the children's rooms to take one last peek. The girls' empty stockings were tied to the foot of their four-poster bed, and Michael's stocking hung from a drawer knob on the bureau in his room. It almost broke my heart. For months, I had been hiding toys in my closet and small surprises to put in their stockings. Would Ben know which treasure to put into each one? I closed the door softly. By the time I had struggled into my coat, Mary Catherine had arrived. Ben was waiting by the front door.

"Let's go," he said nervously, "We have a half hour drive ahead of us."

He helped me to the car. Outside, the brilliance of lights shone from the house windows on our street.

In the car, Ben drove with concentration, asking me every few minutes how I felt.

Ben pulled to a stop in front of the hospital and helped me out of the car. I experienced a hollow feeling of abandonment, like the torn paper and ribbon from the opened boxes on Christmas morning. We had wisely decided that Ben should stay home with the children rather than be with me during the delivery, but I couldn't help but feel sorry for myself. He was going to spend Christmas with the children while I had to spend the holiday alone in the hospital.

By then, it was after midnight. The soft snowfall was heavier now, and the hospital and parking lot were covered in snow. A nurse in the small-town hospital met us at the door and took the suitcase from Ben.

"Mrs. Salata?" the nurse asked. I nodded. "Merry Christmas," she said cheerfully.

I stared at her for a moment, ready to burst into fresh tears. Then the absurdity of her greeting struck me as funny. I began to laugh.

Why should I feel sorry for myself? I thought. *Doctors and nurses had to work on Christmas Eve and other holidays. Thousands of other people couldn't be with their families on special occasions either.*

"Is the maternity ward full?" I asked.

"No," she said. "The doctors discharged their post births. They all wanted to go home for Christmas."

Later, when I had settled in, Ben stooped to kiss me goodbye, promising to remember how much sage to put in the turkey stuffing and which gifts to put in which stockings. Then he turned and swung out the door, blowing me a last kiss.

"Keep your eye on the wall clock," the nurse told me. "Let me know how often the pains are coming. I'll call your doctor when you're ready."

I realized with a shock that I hadn't felt a pain since I'd arrived.

"They've stopped!" I cried. "I should have told my husband to wait. I might be going home tonight."

"That happens sometimes," the nurse said. "But you're going to stay put. You are already overdue. We may have to induce labor."

I slept fitfully through the night. I awoke around seven o'clock Christmas morning, surprised that I had slept so long. *The children have already opened their gifts*, I thought sadly. The knowledge that I could have stayed home until morning, after all, distressed me. *I should have known it would take ages*, I thought. Labor had always been a long, drawn-out affair for me.

The pains started again and were coming at regular intervals. All the other signs of the baby's impending arrival were also apparent. Still, it wasn't until eleven o'clock Christmas night that I was transferred to a gurney and wheeled to the delivery room.

Shortly after midnight, I delivered a beautiful baby boy. I named him Mark, the name Ben and I had chosen.

The next afternoon, Ben came to see me. He kissed me and held me close to him. He thrust a tiny bouquet of flowers into my hands. I buried my nose in their fragrance.

I questioned him eagerly about the children. Had they liked their toys? Did Paula and Kathy's new outfits fit? Were they wearing them?

"I just put some old jeans and sweaters on them," he said sheepishly. "It seemed a whole lot easier."

I closed my eyes, imagining the way things must have been that morning. Paper and ribbons and toys strewn from one end of the room to the other.

"How was your shirt?" I asked. "Does it fit? Do you like it?"

"The shirt?" Ben said. "Oh, the shirt. Sure. It fits perfectly, sweetie. I'm saving it to wear on our next date."

"A plaid shirt?" I teased. "I guess we're not going anywhere special."

"Just kidding," he said with a laugh. "Your mother came over this morning. She's looking after the children. I don't know what I'd do without her."

When Ben kissed me goodbye, I had never felt so forlorn in my life. But the joy of holding and feeding baby Mark made me forget about my lost Christmas.

The next day, Ben was at the hospital early to take us home. The decorations sparkled through the windows of snowy houses framing the road like scenes from old-fashioned Christmas cards. But for me, Christmas had vanished like a department store Santa.

Ben swung the car off the road and turned into the driveway of our red brick house. I could see three small faces pressed against the window. Ben took baby Mark out in his car seat as I hurried into the house. My mother stood in the doorway, and we hugged and kissed each other as I entered. The children jumped up and down, hugging me warmly and smothering me with kisses.

"Where's Mark?" they shouted. "Where's our new baby?"

Ben came in and placed the baby in his car seat carefully on the floor in front of the children. Michael, Kathy, and Paula exclaimed over their new baby brother as they gathered around him like three small magi worshipping the Baby Jesus.

I stopped in the doorway of the living room and withdrew a sharp breath.

The tree stood in the corner exactly the way it had looked on Christmas Eve. Underneath, instead of the unwrapped presents I had expected, the unopened gifts were stacked neatly, their silver bows and shiny ribbons intact.

"I don't understand," I whispered. "Nothing has been opened yet."

"We saved Christmas for you, honey," Ben said softly, putting his arm around me. His eyes shone with love and tenderness.

"You waited for me?" was all I could say. "You saved Christmas for me."

"We waited! We waited!" Paula sang, dancing up and down. "We've been practicing carols, and there's a turkey in the oven."

"Can we open our presents now?" Michael wanted to know.

"Let's gather around the tree," Ben said. He looked at my mother. "Grandma, do you want to play Santa Claus?"

I sat within the circle of my family, watching the children open the glittering gifts one by one. I heard them laugh and exclaim over the games, toys, and clothes. I realized, yet again, that the spirit of Christmas is in giving and, even more important, in sharing with one another.

In waiting to share their holiday celebration with me, my family gave me the next-best Christmas gift I've ever received. The very best was my almost-Christmas baby, Mark.

—*Estelle Salata*

Baby Makes Four

When I was a child, I was not enamored with babies. An only child to the bone, I found small children irritating, and babies, with their perpetual drooling and persistent diaper odor, were the worst. My mother and other adults would point out cute specimens, hoping to pique my interest, but I promptly turned up my nose at each one. This trickled down even to my play habits. The idea of playing house was enough to send me running to climb the highest tree in sight.

Animals were different. I cherished my stuffed animals as much as I detested dolls. I might twist the head off a Barbie, but I would swaddle a stuffed bear and rock it to sleep. I loved the real things, too; there wasn't a kitty, puppy, hamster, fish, or canary alive that I didn't want to "mommy" and play with. Even as a teen and into my early twenties, I would pick a golden retriever over a cute baby any day.

My first child was a Himalayan cat named Margot. She filled the emptiness of my graduate school apartment and life. I adored her and turned into one of those crazy pet people, putting her picture in frames around the house and dressing her up for Halloween. My cat was my baby, and I was her mommy. She was a snuggly sort of cat, so I carried her around the house with me and let her sleep on my bed. She was the perfect child—sweet and loving without the upkeep.

Time tempered my aversion to babies, and as a young woman, although I didn't actually gravitate toward them, they no longer repulsed me either. Despite my earlier heebie-jeebies about babies, I started thinking about having a family someday, and I convinced myself that maybe things would be different with my own children. In fact, I was banking on the idea that motherhood is somehow innate, that we naturally know how to care for our own young. I certainly didn't have any practical experience.

After I was married, my feline child didn't suffice for long, and I became pregnant. It was a planned thing, and I was excited. Still, I was apprehensive. What if motherhood wasn't for me? What if I was better suited to cleaning out a litter box? My friends reassured me that I would be fine, that I was very maternal with Margot. I didn't believe them, and I'm not sure they were convinced themselves. After all, cats and babies are not at all the same thing. I worried that I would prefer my cat to my child. Margot was so soft and adorable. It was a tough act to follow.

As it turned out, I was right about motherhood being innate—for me, at least. When my daughter, Justine, was born, it was the most natural thing in the world for me to care for her. The drooling, the pooping, the strange smells—what was disgusting in others I found delightful in her. I held her competently and comfortably, immediately, as though I had been holding babies my whole life. Holding kitties and puppies hadn't been bad practice, after all. My first diaper change was a little bumpy, but I was a quick study and a week later, I doubt an outsider would have noticed the difference between my technique and any experienced mother's.

When it came time to bring Justine home from the hospital, I finally remembered my "other" child. Strange how she had slipped my mind for a few days. Other pet owners advised us to have the pet's primary caretaker walk into the home alone, while the other parent held the baby, to help ease the transition for the pet. So, my husband carried Justine in her infant carrier, and I opened the door to greet Margot.

I had been so preoccupied with my own motherhood worries that I hadn't really given much thought to this new, quasi-sibling relationship. My fears shifted from Margot's well-being to Justine's. I hoped that Margot would be accepting and, above all, not aggressive. Now, it was clear that if things didn't go well, she would be the one to go. I hoped my children could at least coexist, if not love each other.

Margot didn't hiss at Justine. She didn't hide under the nearest couch. Nor did she seek refuge in my arms. Rather, she did what I didn't believe a cat was capable of doing—she understood. She sat at an interested but safe distance from Justine. She looked from me to the infant carrier and back to me again. Things had changed forever, and she was aware of it.

Once I realized what was happening, I rushed to my fluffy child and gathered her in my arms. "Oh, Margot," I blubbered into her fur. "Mommy loves you, too. You are still a part of this family." Margot looked impassively at me, as if to say, We'll see. She knew then what I didn't understand until later—that in that moment, she had become a cat again.

Margot is still my beloved pet, but I'm not really her mommy anymore. Occasionally, I'll still refer to myself as my cat's "Mommy" out of habit, but the word tastes strange in my mouth. Someone else owns that relationship, and it's not so easy to give away now. Margot, in conversation, is now "the cat." She may be the best cat in the world, but a cat she is, and my "baby" is someone else.

Justine, mercifully, did not inherit my early dislike of babies. She loves them, excitedly pointing out any she sees. She shares my love for animals, though. She's an equal opportunity nurturer, caring for dolls and stuffed animals alike. Her favorite animal of all is Margot, who has been renamed "Mow," because that's the sound she makes.

Mow herself is a study in patience, and if there are candidates for animal sainthood, I'd like to nominate her. She has stoically endured rough hands, tail pullings, and countless clumsy kisses. She even allows herself to be lugged through the house like a sack of potatoes. I'd like to think that she does it out of love for my daughter, but I can see with every stare in my direction that it is out of loyalty to me.

I now believe that mothers come from all different paths of life. The lifelong babysitter is not necessarily more qualified than someone who has never held a baby. Nurturing is practiced in all sorts of different ways; for some it may be caring for a little sister, for others it may be tending a garden. Though I didn't know it then, throughout my entire life I had been training for motherhood. For me, taking care of my stuffed animals and later my cat was all the experience I needed to become a loving and devoted mother to my daughter.

—*Amanda Callendrier*

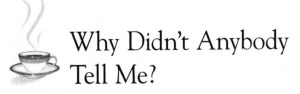

Why Didn't Anybody Tell Me?

I can only imagine how pitiful I looked wandering the halls of the maternity ward, my belly in the lead, portable IV in tow, a woman on a desperate mission.

An older lady passed and smiled. "Don't worry, hon. You'll have that baby any minute."

She was gone before I managed to get out, "But . . . I had her yesterday."

It was true. I didn't look much different than I had when I checked into the hospital. But that was just fluid, right?

I finally found what I'd been hunting: a scale. Gingerly, I hoisted up one foot and then the other. My eyes fixed on the numbers in front of me as I inched the metal weights from left to right—and stared in horror. Was this someone's idea of a joke? I delivered an eight-pound baby sixteen hours ago.

Shouldn't I have lost at least eight pounds? Why didn't anybody tell me about this?

I'd heard a plethora of unsolicited advice during my pregnancy. I heard all about sleepless nights, stretch marks, night sweats, and (*gasp!*) cracked nipples. Why hadn't someone slipped in a little something like, "Look, you'll get as big as Jackie Gleason, go to the hospital, have the baby, and go home two days later still looking nine months pregnant."

I'd been subjected to every horrifying story of women delivering at home, breech births, miscarriages, and still births. Total strangers had approached me in restaurants and offered explicit details about passing their mucous plugs. (What?) For some reason, when other women noticed I was pregnant, hemorrhoids, placentas, and meconium stools became acceptable subjects of conversation. Apparently, they were certain I'd be interested in hearing how they "tore while delivering the twins," but figured a minor detail like having to wear maternity clothes to the baby's one-month check up wouldn't interest me.

No one was less prepared than I was for this or the many other surprises I found waiting for me as a new mom. Why didn't anybody tell me, when they were singing the praises of breastfeeding, that it's a guessing game at best, that you can read all the nursing books in all the bookstores from Atlanta to Alaska, and you'll still find yourself sitting bleary-eyed at 4:00 A.M. with a wailing baby in your arms, wondering, *Was it the tomato sauce? Should I cut out dairy? Caffeine? Chocolate?*

Why didn't anyone tell me, when they were all offering free babysitting, that one look at this glorious creature and I wouldn't trust my own mother to watch her? I'd read articles about husbands feeling jealous of the time their wives devote to the baby. No one prepared me for the first time after Haley's birth when David and I were feeling (shall we say) romantic, and he whispered, "You're a good mommy." "Good mommy" wasn't what I was going for.

I'd heard plenty about terrible twos, temper tantrums, and time-outs. No one told me I'd gladly throw myself in front of a speeding train to save my daughter but that I would also lie awake at night imagining all the horrible things that might happen to me before I had the chance to watch her grow up.

Someone might have prepared me for the desperate night when I tore through my parenting books in search of a chapter on how to get rid of colic, only to find instead, "Learning to Live with Colic." Live with it? Why would I want to live with it?

When I bought a secondhand saxophone, thinking I'd need a hobby to fill up all those hours when the baby was sleeping, someone might have explained just how full my days would become.

When I talked about how I'd feed her, bathe her, and put her to sleep, but didn't know what I'd do with the rest of my day, they might have described to me a day like today, when it's 12:00 noon and I'm wondering whether I'll ever find time to get out of my jammies, much less take a shower.

Surely, someone could have told me not to call 911 when she choked on water, that it would gush from the bottle like Old Faithful. And it would have been nice for someone other than my pediatrician to reassure me that the lump on the side of her tiny neck is not a cancerous tumor, but a normal, healthy lymph gland.

They might have mentioned how lonely I'd get when I put my career on hold to stay home and be the world's best mom. That one day I'd find myself feeling so isolated I'd corner the meter reader in the driveway and subject him to every excruciating detail of a day at home with the baby. That I'd be so ravenous for adult conversation I'd watch the clock, praying for 6:00 when my husband came home from work, and then pounce on him the second he walked through the door, talking a mile a minute about nothing and everything and anything.

Why didn't anybody tell me how different my life would be? And how difficult some of it can be?

Yet, as I look at this amazing little person who shared my body for nine months, this much I know for sure: I'd gain 100 pounds, give up lattes for life, redefine my relationship with my husband, abandon my career for good, and never get another good night's sleep to be the mama she deserves. I've just got one more question: What exactly do I do with this belly button thing when it finally falls off?

—*Mimi Greenwood Knight*

The Wisdom Well

Falling pregnant. That's the British term for this most dramatic and miraculous event. As though you aren't minding your step and suddenly stumble over a cliff and fall, with your body ballooning up as rapidly as it plummets. I understood the term at age thirty-seven when I "fell pregnant," never having really planned for children and certainly not so soon after being swept off my feet into an equally unplanned marriage.

My hazy understanding was that pregnancy meant swollen ankles, hemorrhoids, indigestion (if one were lucky enough to want to look at food), and above all—fat, fat, fat. I had never experienced a friend's pregnancy secondhand, and I'd never had the opportunity for my mother to share her pregnancy experiences with me, as she died when I was twenty. When I fell pregnant, I had been in the Middle East for five years and I was working with the Jerusalem office of UNICEF. Many of my local friends were younger and single; those internationals closer to my age were free and unencumbered. Friends at home were getting on with their careers; the few with children might have bought them at the corner store for all I had heard about their pregnancies.

From the moment I realized I was going to have a baby, I felt simply wonderful—well, after the amazing sleep patterns passed, of course. For the first few weeks, I spent far more time horizontal and snoring than upright and intelligible. Every afternoon at about 3:30, Mr. Sandman would wield a baseball bat that sent me off into a deep sleep. Nothing and nobody could keep me awake. I would sleep until about 8:30 in the evening, wake up, eat something, and go immediately back to bed to sleep soundly the rest of the night.

Then, when I was about ten weeks along, the fatigue just melted away, and I was on top of the world. I was flooded with energy and high spirits. I ate heartily but well, my only downfall being that the local ice cream company, Rukab's, had a multitude of cooler-carrying vendors who seemed magically to cross my path half a dozen times a day. People told me I was glowing, and I could see it. I felt beautiful, and for the first time since before my teen years, I was at peace with my body. I realized how ridiculous my American preoccupation with weight was when the sanctioned weight gain of pregnancy gave me an unprecedented sense of freedom. That heavy burden had been my constant companion for over two decades, and I hadn't even been aware of it. Once it was gone, I felt like Bambi, "twitter-pated."

In the midst of my joy, however, I also felt loneliness. I wished for my mother with an immediacy that suggested an absence of twenty days rather than almost twenty years. I felt as though the change in my life and the changes in my body had set me apart, placed me in a joyous, yet separate, space. It was as though I were in a golden bubble looking out at the world.

Telephone lines could be quite difficult to obtain, particularly in rented properties, and I had lived for almost five years without a phone at home. For the most part, it had never bothered me. If there was anything urgent, I used the telephone at work, and my family could always reach me there, if needed. The time difference between California and the Middle East was not conducive to regular chatting, and I longed to share my experience with someone, to be welcomed into the inner circle of maternity. Sitting in my obstetrician's waiting room, people tended to stare a bit at first and then turn back to their own companions. Although there were friendly smiles, none of the chatter was extended to include me, and I didn't seem able to bridge the gap and reach these knowledgeable women who, conditioned by tradition and culture, took child-bearing in stride.

Wafa, a woman at work, told me of the delivery of her first child, and I listened to her tale of unbearable pain and endless screams that carried over into her dreams. I wondered whether this would feel relevant to me at some point in the future, but I could not believe it would be. So I listened and sympathized, and left her tale behind me when I left the office that day.

I thought of my mother again and how not being able to share my pregnancy with her deprived me of the reassurance of knowing what pregnancy had been like for her. Surely, her experiences would apply to me, as her genetic legatee.

I confided in Laura, a comfortable, knowledgeable midwife who worked with UNICEF. Her knowledge seemed to rest with her, however. She remained the generous source and I the naïve country girl with the empty jug. When would I, too, grow large and comfortable with the knowledge that came with childbearing?

Despite the lack of other mothers with whom I could compare notes, for the most part I sailed along confident in my beauty, in love with my body and its vital processes. I was living a miracle and felt gifted.

One night I was sitting up in bed, looking down at my modest but sizeable bump, imagining the baby girl inside, and suddenly, panic struck. My mind fast-forwarded to the delivery room, completely overriding any blissful imaginings of what my daughter would be like once she was no longer within my body. The thought of birthing and then caring for this tiny human being entrusted to my care filled me with terror, and I was overcome with the sensation of being on a rollercoaster ride from which I could not now escape. A sound like rushing air filled my ears, and my breath came in short, panting spurts. When I turned to my husband, Allan, and told him how I was feeling, he brushed it aside as being "silly," saying dismissively, "You just can't think like that." Clearly, he was uncomfortable with the feelings I was expressing and did not know how to help; it was easier to simply reject them.

Then a feeling of calm came over me as I reminded myself that millions of other women had been down this path before me and that my body would naturally alter to accommodate childbirth, a process far older than me. I envisioned this huge, reassuring procession of women, one by one doing their part and passing along the wisdom to ensure the continuing cycle of humanity. It occurred to me that I was now part of that infinite chain of mothers, linked soul to soul, birth to birth. As my breathing slowed, I saw myself stepping off the rollercoaster and joining the procession. I felt in harmony with generations of women and as though I had passed an important initiation test. (Achieving calm accep-tance that a basketball-sized baby is going to pass through a hole in my body the size of a dime is a pretty challenging initiation test!) The next morning I felt different. I was ready—to give birth and to take on all that meant.

Several days later, we had a visit from Ruth, a Kenyan woman who worked with an international Christian aid agency that was supporting the agricultural development project Allan was working on. We had become friendly with her over the course of several visits to the project, and she had been over for dinner once or twice. Now, she had a young woman with her, whom she introduced as Beatrice, her niece.

Beatrice was healthily rounded, abundantly plump all over—and pregnant. She was about seven months along, and her bump was huge and high. I could feel my eyes continually exploring her abdomen, which seemed enormous, compared with mine, even though I was almost to my due date.

Beatrice's moon-shaped face seemed made for smiles, and her large brown eyes twinkled with humor, despite her circumstances and youth. Just eighteen, she had fallen in love with a married man and had an affair with him. Her family knew nothing of the relationship until she fell pregnant and was rejected by her lover. Then, desperately embarrassed and anxious to remove her from their small town, they shipped Beatrice off to stay with her aunt in Jerusalem, until the gossip—and her bump—had faded away.

We chatted, and I asked Beatrice how she was enjoying her visit. Her answers were accompanied by smiles and laughter, and she seemed older than her age, comfortable and relaxed, despite having been banished from the bosom of her family. She was so colorful in her dress, looks, and personality that I marveled at her vibrancy and confidence.

Ruth and Allan became engrossed in a discussion of work, and I went to make tea. Beatrice offered to help and followed me through to our tiny kitchen. She had seemed to be as fascinated with me as I was with her, and her large dark eyes kept straying to my tiny bump, my reddish hair, my freckles. We chatted as the water boiled, and I prepared the kettle with loose tea, exchanging due dates and other details of our condition.

Beatrice then fell silent, and when I looked over at her, she was looking down. Then she turned to me, her eyes huge and pleading, and she suddenly seemed very much her age, nearly twenty years younger than me, and in disgrace, far from home, and pregnant.

"Aren't you scared?" she asked. "I am so scared. I wonder what will happen, and I am afraid of the pain."

I placed my hand gently on her arm. "Do you feel that you are going downhill very fast and you can't stop?" I asked her.

She looked shocked, like I had somehow reached inside her mind and plucked out her thoughts. I told her how I had felt that evening some nights before and how I had reached a state of relaxation and what I had told myself, and I sensed that my words were easing her mind. I felt her breaking through the fear barrier and her spirit moving toward me, as we shared the wisdom women have shared through the ages, across generations, across national, cultural, and political boundaries. As we drew our water from the same source, I could feel that my jug was no longer empty and that we were no longer standing alone. We were now both part of a great and grand procession, cheering and waving and creating a loud and joyful noise in the world.

—*Rose-Marie Barbeau*

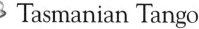 Tasmanian Tango

Shortly after Gregory was born, the doctor placed him on my chest, positioning him to feed. Gregory opened his mouth wide. I expected him to latch onto my breast and begin sucking. Instead, he wailed with all of his might and resisted my breast, arching his back and flailing his arms, with surprising strength for a one-hour-old. Such chaos is not how I had pictured my first attempt at breastfeeding, because none of the photos of nursing mommies I'd seen featured a hysterical baby. Parenting how-to books with illustrations of serene mothers nursing angelic babies led me to believe that breastfeeding would happen naturally. Nursing mommy memoirs and articles about breastfeeding bliss in parenting magazines made no mention of the reality that breastfeeding may not be instinctive for mother or child.

I pressed the red call button on my hospital bed.

A nurse came and gave me a quick (and the operative word here is "quick") lesson in Breastfeeding 101. "You must introduce your baby to your breast," she explained before leaving me alone with my still-wailing and still-not-latching-on infant son.

I held my breast with one hand and flapped it up and down in front of Gregory's face. "Hello there, Gregory. Nice to meet you," I said in a Kermit the Frog voice. His hair-raising scream made it very clear that he had no interest in meeting my breasts. I needed a different approach.

I called for another nurse. This one came with a baby doll for demonstrating proper breastfeeding technique. "Just shove your breast in your baby's mouth while he's crying," she advised, as she palmed the doll's head like Shaquille O'Neal would a basketball and rammed the doll's face into her chest. I winced at hearing the thud, but I was ready. No more Mrs. Nice Mommy.

When Gregory started to cry, I shoved his head to my breast. The harder he cried, the harder I shoved. We went back and forth, crying and shoving, shoving and crying, until we were both just crying.

Neither the no-nonsense nor the neighborly approach to breastfeeding worked, and the nurses' conflicting advice confused and distressed me. I searched through my parenting books again, ignoring the pictures and reading intently for any information about troubleshooting breastfeeding problems. The problems I came across, however, were problems that I wished I had: sore nipples from breastfeeding, baby bites while breastfeeding, baby won't wean from the breast. What do I do if my baby won't breastfeed in the first place?

My husband was clueless. My mother had no breastfeeding experience. I didn't want to call any of my friends who had children, because I was too ashamed to admit that I couldn't do what was supposed to come naturally.

Since my mothering instincts were seemingly nonexistent, I relied on other skills to see me through. I'm a consultant by profession, so I decided to tackle my breastfeeding problem as I would a problem that fell outside my area of expertise for a client: I hired another consultant to solve it for me. Joan, a La Leche League consultant, came to my house to witness the Tasmanian Tango I had come to know as breastfeeding—flailing arms, kicking legs, and lots of screaming. Joan recommended that we keep trying, but in the meantime, I should feed Gregory my expressed milk with a finger-feeder, a plastic bottle with a long, thin straw attached to it, which I taped to my index finger. Gregory drew milk from the straw by sucking on my finger. I felt silly using the finger feeder, like I was nursing a sick baby bird, but I would have tried breastfeeding upside down in the shower if it would have helped.

"Forget the myth that breastfeeding comes easily to a mother and baby," Joan assured me. "Many women struggle with it."

Knowing that I was not alone didn't make me feel any better at three o'clock in the morning while my nipples were squeezed into the plastic suction cups of an electric pump. For the next four weeks, I would pump, do the Tasmanian Tango, and then use the finger feeder, leaving me just enough time to pee before starting the routine all over again. Pump. Tango. Finger Feed. Pump. Tango. Finger Feed. . . . I was beginning to think that keeping Gregory alive might kill me.

I called Joan in tears, "I'm exhausted! I don't know if it's even worth trying anymore."

"Welcome to parenthood," Joan replied. "You're going to feel like that many more times in your life."

While Joan's response wasn't the "there, there" pat on the back I was expecting, it made me view my situation in a new light. Rather than deem my inability to breastfeed as an indictment on my motherly instincts, I decided to view it as training for future challenges I would encounter as a parent. I recommitted myself to trying. I still cried when Gregory kicked and screamed at my breast, but I told myself that if Gregory never breastfeeds, it won't be because I gave up.

One morning six weeks after Gregory was born, I gently pushed his head to my breast. He didn't cry. He didn't kick. Miraculously, he began sucking my nipple and didn't stop until he was full. There's been no more Tasmanian Tango. Still, while breastfeeding is now easy and enjoyable, I can say from first-hand experience that it was not at all "intuitive." In fact, I'm pretty sure the only thing about motherhood that comes naturally is to feel like a failure if your baby isn't crawling, walking, or drinking from a sippy cup in sync with the "My Baby This Week" e-mail alerts. But the next time I feel like I'm failing as a mother, I will look at Gregory's finger feeder and remember that he and I can overcome most challenges as long as we don't stop trying.

—Elizabeth Ridley

Picking up the Stitches

My childhood memories hold images of my mother, always knitting. I can recall her sitting in waiting rooms, by the pool, or on our sofa, with iridescent colored needles looped in yarn clicking away between her hands. She knit in European fashion, the way her mother had taught her: left index finger held straight up, wrapped in yarn to control the tension of the stitches. She'd spin that finger in circles at regular intervals, counterclockwise to release the yarn into the piece she was knitting, clockwise to pull additional yarn from the skein by her side.

When I was seven, she taught me to knit. I sat in the cocoon of her warmth, nestled on the couch beside her, while she cast on a small row of stitches and demonstrated how to insert the tip of the needle into the ring of yarn and pull it out and over, catching and pulling through the loop the string of yarn held taut by the extended finger. I knit a headband. My meager creation with its all-knit pattern paled in comparison to my mother's work. Next, she taught me the more difficult purl stitch, and I worked on a ribbed scarf. She expertly picked up and wove back through my lost stitches. Eventually, I completed a lavender and yellow scarf too amateurish to wear.

Winter after winter, my sister and I wore our mother's hand-knit sweaters—the winter white, fisherman-type pullovers with their thick cables; the smooth, stocking stitch, button-down cardigans with raglan sleeves. As young as we were, we recognized the love and care that went into each creation. I remember one year, in a minor sledding collision, the runners of the opposing sled somehow getting up under my jacket and snagging my sweater. At home, I stared at the ripped yarn, the jagged hole torn through my mother's hard work, and hid the sweater at the bottom of a dresser drawer. A few months later, after she'd repeatedly asked why I didn't wear that particular sweater, I finally had the courage to show it to her.

Shortly after that, my mother had to stop knitting. Her fingers, stiff and swollen with rheumatoid arthritis, couldn't manage the dexterous movements. At first she decreased her productivity, knitting fewer hours each day, but pain and medical advice eventually convinced her to give it up entirely. I have since heard different theories, that using the joints actually retains their mobility, but in those days her doctor advised her to discontinue knitting, so she did.

Over the years, she occasionally mentioned in passing, especially when buying our winter clothes, how she missed knitting. It wasn't until I was pregnant with her first grandchild, however, that she truly lamented the loss.

"I wish I could knit for the baby," she said early into my pregnancy, before I'd even begun to show.

"It's okay, Mom," I reassured her. "They sell lovely knit items in the store."

"It's not the same. A baby should have something handmade." Her voice drifted off, and then she added wistfully, "I wish I hadn't given away all those things I knitted when you were a baby."

My mother has a strong sense of tradition. She's passed down to me a powerful system of beliefs and values, along with some odd superstitions and family customs. But she's also a pragmatic and generous person who'd passed along our outgrown sweaters, painstakingly and carefully knit, to friends and relatives with younger children. Now, she regretted that decision.

Call it a product of the nesting instinct, call it a growing awareness of my mom's definition of tradition, but in my sixth month, a vague, subconscious inkling that had been budding during my pregnancy became a clear, conscious longing. My fingers itched to create something, stitch by loving stitch, with a definable shape from a loose tangle of yarn. It turned out that my mother, who had given away the products of her knitting labor, still had all the supplies. From deep in her closet she pulled out a box filled with aluminum needles in various lengths, thicknesses, and colors, just as I'd remembered them—iridescent golds and purples, greens and blues, each numbered needle assigned its own hue. There were cable hooks, circular and double-pointed needles, plus, believe it or not, leftover yarn. She also had her old pattern books. At first glance, the books were outdated, the sweaters modeled by men, women, and children with late 1950s and early 1960s pants and hairdos, everything photographed in black-and-white. But closer inspection revealed many of the sweater styles to be timeless.

"Take it, take it all," my mother said, meeting my renewed childhood interest with an eager thrust of the repacked box into my waiting arms.

At home, I made a slipknot a few feet into the loose end of a string of yarn and tightened it around a knitting needle. My fingers remembered what I'd been shown so many years before, how to stretch the yarn from each side of the slipknot between the thumb and index finger of my left hand, twisting, looping and tightening, casting on the starter row. I wrapped a few rings of wool around my extended left finger, inserted the right needle into the front of the first cast-on stitch, and began to knit.

It took me a month to knit a yellow-and-white striped baby blanket, a boxy knit-purl pattern I made up myself. Between the thick yarn I'd bought and the number ten needles I used, the work went quickly. My mother watched its progress in silence, commenting once I finished that it was a bit bulky to wrap around a baby.

My next project was a white baby sweater with a matching hat, knit from the finest, softest yarn on thin, number two needles. It was the first time I'd followed a pattern, increased or decreased stitches, or sewed together seams. I finished two months later, timed perfectly a few days shy of my due date, marveling that it had taken me longer to complete a project about a tenth the size of my previous one. My mother overlooked the unevenness in the tension of the stitches, reflected in the waviness of the bottom hem and the crimped front edge where I sewed tiny pearl buttons, pronouncing it absolutely suitable for a baby to wear.

And then the baby was late.

Bored and restless, I looked through the box my mother had so eagerly given me months before, leafing through the many pattern books. Some were older than I'd originally thought; indeed, the copyright dates for most of the men's and women's books were the early- to mid-fifties, before my sister or I had been born. It occurred to me that although I recalled my father wearing a few vests that my mother had knit for him, I had never seen her knit for anyone other than my sister and me, with the exception of the occasional baby gift.

When I called to ask her about this, she said, "Children's stuff was smaller and quicker to knit." I believed her until, years later, looking back on all the sweaters I'd knit with such meticulous care for my own three children, which they so carelessly spit up on as babies and dirtied as toddlers and then quickly outgrew, I realized that small and quick had nothing to do with it. It was about the endurance of love, not the practicality of use.

So a week overdue and too uncomfortable to browse through the stores, I picked out a simple cardigan pattern from one of my mother's books and some skeins of her leftover yarn, and started to knit. I became obsessed with finishing the sweater before I went into labor, and a week or so later, my wrist sore from the constant, repetitive motion, it was done.

"What yarn are you using?" my mother asked during one of her daily are-you-in-labor-yet phone calls.

"The only one there was enough of," I said. "It's maroon."

"Maroon!" She couldn't have sounded more shocked had I told her I was having triplets. "Maroon is not a color for a baby."

I brought my first baby, my mother's first grand-daughter, home from the hospital a few days later, wearing the delicate white hat and sweater set, wrapped in the bulky yellow-and-white striped blanket. She never wore the maroon sweater. In my inexperience, I'd knit it for a six-month-old. She turned six months old in June.

Neither of my other two children wore that maroon baby sweater either. By the time they came along, I had learned enough as a mother to know my own mother had been right: Not only was maroon the wrong color for a baby, but the short button-less sweater I'd knit with its long tie around the neck was the wrong shape and style as well. Twenty-two years later, it's still tucked away, along with the blankets and sweaters I made for my three children while they were young, in a box in the back of my closet.

My mother's knitting supplies are stored in my basement, along with the pattern books and needles I purchased over the years, deposited for safekeeping when the demands of three growing children cur-tailed my knitting. There are also a few saved skeins of leftover yarn in various textures and colors, including enough maroon for a headband, ready for the next generation to pick them up.

—*Peggy Duffy*

The Procedure

I sip herbal tea, staring out the kitchen window, soaking in the beauty of our backyard. In the middle of a lush hill of ivy, an old California oak rises—a perfect host for a tree house, one that someday will be built for the baby I'm carrying. I'm only three months pregnant, but already, Brian and I are excited about being parents. I place the teacup in the sink, grab my purse, and head for my second appointment with Dr. R.

My OB-GYN leans against the pink linoleum countertop in a sterile examination room. Fluorescent lights buzz as she folds her thin, pale arms across her chest. She frowns. "You're not interested?"

I smile and look deep into her stern eyes, trying to connect. I am hoping that because she's a woman and only a few years older than me she will understand my position. "I know this sounds odd," I explain, "but I feel like a young thirty-eight. I was a late bloomer. And I'm very healthy. My intuition tells me the baby's fine and I don't really need this. But you're the expert. Do you think the amniocentesis is absolutely necessary?" I'm rambling, but I can't help it. This doctor inspires nervousness.

Dr. R tilts her head and stares at me. Her frown lines grow deeper. "Well, Cheryl, you are thirty-eight, even if you don't feel it, and we don't want to take any chances now, do we? Yes, having the amnio is the wise choice."

She's straightforward; I like that. I mean, I think I do. My girlfriend Bonnie recommended Dr. R. She liked her sense of humor—which I've yet to see—and her no-nonsense approach, which made Bonnie feel cared for. Frankly, I feel bullied. I wish Brian were here, but I didn't see any need to pull him away from his work for this visit. Still, Bonnie did deliver two healthy babies. And Dr. R is so confident of the need for the amnio. Plus, my mother and most of my friends share her belief. I give in. I'll have the procedure.

Dr. R half-smiles approvingly and then orders me to book an appointment at the front desk. "See you in five weeks," she says brusquely as she sweeps out of the room.

I forget all about Dr. R's cool behavior as the days fly by. We whirl right through the holiday season, and in a blink, it's the first Thursday in January, time for the procedure. Brian and I have taken the morning off work. I feel calm, confident, and centered. That's what I chant as Brian and I drive on the congested freeway toward Santa Monica in a downpour. It's been raining since we left home, and watching the raindrops collect at the base of the car window, I wonder if we'll ever reach the west side.

My friend Joan is meeting us at the office. I chose Joan for support because her nurturing demeanor makes me feel safe and loved, always.

"Nervous?" Brian asks, inching forward in the traffic.

"Not at all," I say with all the confidence I can muster. "Why should I be? Everyone says it's a breeze." I don't mention the butterflies swarming in the pit of my stomach—the result, I assume, of my excitement at the notion that'll we'll soon learn our baby's gender.

"Not at all?" Brian prods.

I shake my head, pushing aside all fears, especially the one about the needle that will soon go straight through my abdomen into my uterus.

We arrive on time and walk arm-in-arm into the five-story medical building. I spot Joan sitting in the waiting room reading a detective novel; she loves those. She stands and embraces both of us. The receptionist hands me a sheaf of papers, and I fill in blanks while Brian and Joan discuss the weather. Minutes later, a no-nonsense nurse ushers us into a windowless examination room tinier than a storage closet. I'd pictured something large and bright. Where are the fresh flowers and cheery pictures?

Joan sits on a stool in the corner, while Brian stands in the changing area, which is partially veiled by a shabby curtain. I hoist myself onto the examination table, which seems enormous since it takes up most of the space. The room is freezing. I pull my leather coat tightly around me and wait for further instructions.

Finally, the nurse enters and with not so much as a hello, slaps down on the counter two pairs of rubber gloves, extracts an enormous needle from a cupboard, and unfurls a blood pressure gauge and wraps it around my arm, where goose bumps begin to crawl. Before I can even ask for the blood pressure numbers, she's out the door. A few seconds later, she pops her head in one more time.

"Oh by the way, the doctor will be detained about forty-five minutes."

"What?" Brian blurts.

"She's delivering," the nurse says flatly.

"What, flowers?" Brian asks, trying to lighten the gloomy mood.

"A baby," the nurse says sternly, then catching on, giggles and adds, "Don't worry, she shouldn't be any longer than that. I mean, all she really has to do is stand there and catch the baby."

With that, she vanishes.

Joan looks at me, I look at her, and we both look at Brian.

"This is ridiculous," I say.

"What, honey?" Joan asks as if talking to a disappointed child.

"This," I spread my arms, but I'm not sure what I mean. "You need a stool, Bri. I'll go get one." I hop off the table and rush down the antiseptic hall to the nurse's station, where my nurse is swapping stories with two others.

"Um, excuse me," I say politely, "may I have an extra stool—for my husband?"

She shakes her head no. "Sorry. Fire hazard in a room that size; no can do."

No can do? I slink back to my room.

I shrug as I enter what now feels like my cell. "No can do," I repeat.

"Listen, Cheryl," Joan says gently, "I'll go sit in the waiting room. I have my book. Just call me when you want me."

I nod dejectedly. Brian, needing to call his clients to let them know he'll be detained, follows her. I watch them both exit, and then, alone in the miniscule room, stare at the needle, the gloves, the dirty pink walls. When Brian returns, we stare together.

After what seems an eternity, Dr. R walks in and nods. I introduce her to Brian. She dutifully shakes his hand.

"All right, Cheryl," she says. "Lay back, put your feet in the stirrups, pull your pants down and your shirt up." She's like a drill sergeant.

Naturally, I obey. The stirrups are as chilly as her manner.

"You should have been scheduled on a Tuesday. That's when the ultrasound technician is in. I don't actually do a full ultrasound. You'll have to come back for that." All the while, she's squirting cold jelly on my abdomen and moving the ultrasound scanner from one side of it to the other.

"This is a small screen," she sighs. "Brian, stand over here, and I'll turn off the lights so you can see your baby on the screen."

I sit propped up on my elbows so I can see, too.

"See that pulsing in the middle?" Both of us move closer and squint. "That's the heart."

The picture is a blur. I want to see my baby's spine. I want to see hands and feet. I'm disappointed. Still, we can see our baby's heart beating, and that's something. Something wonderful.

I smile at Brian as my eyes well with tears. I'm ready now. I take a deep breath. Dr. R snaps on rubber gloves, scans my belly again, and marks a black X on my lower abdomen. Out of the corner of my eye I notice Brain is back on his stool—head in hands. Needles make him queasy.

The nurse hands the doctor the needle; I inhale again and feel a pinch. *That wasn't so bad,* I think. But apparently, that wasn't the needle. Without warning, with no time for another breath, the doctor stabs my belly and I feel drawing pain, then searing cramps.

"Wow, I felt that," I gasp. The cramps intensify. "It hurts," I whisper as tears flow down my face. My insides feel as though they're being sucked up through the needle.

"Stop!" I howl, "Please." I beg.

My body is rigid with pain. I have nothing to hold onto. The nurse doesn't offer her hand, I can't reach the doctor, and Brian is probably passed out. I clutch at air, my back tensing into an arch.

"I can't take anymore," I whimper.

"Almost done," Dr. R says, withdrawing the needle.

The doctor and nurse exchange a look. The cramps are easing, but the pain remains. I'm panting as the nurse hurries out of the room.

Dr. R is scribbling on her clipboard as she moves toward me. "I think you should come back on Tuesday," she says.

"What do you mean?"

"We have to do this again," she crosses those arrogant arms. "I didn't get the fluid."

Blood rushes to my head. "You hurt me like that and you didn't even get the fluid?" I scream.

"Unfortunately, we didn't get that far."

Escorted by the nurse, Joan enters, takes one look at me, and begins stroking my head. I'm shaking uncontrollably, but Dr. R is still talking.

"I don't want to try this again today. It might be too much."

"You think?" I scream.

Dr. R leans against the counter. I stare at her chenille sweater, at the green matching floral skirt. I focus in on mother-of-pearl buttons.

"Better still," she says, scribbling, "Let's send you to a specialist."

Now my blood doesn't just rush, it boils. "Everyone said this was such a breeze, and now I need a specialist?" I hiss.

Joan massages my shoulders. "Cheryl, honey, maybe a specialist would be better."

Then she spots Brian in the corner and motions him to follow her out of the room to get some air. Pale and unable to speak, he trails behind her.

I turn to the doctor. "You hurt me," I accuse.

"Cheryl, sometimes the uterus contracts. We had to put the needle in a sensitive area because of the baby's position."

"Well, you might have warned me, instead of just—drilling for oil."

She shrugs. "It's different for everyone."

She hands me the specialist's card and walks out of the room.

When she is gone, I lie there, flummoxed, and start to cry again—ashamed and blaming myself for choosing this cold, unfeeling doctor. I dress slowly. My belly throbs. I blow my nose, wipe away tears, and then, each step deliberate so I don't increase the pain, I walk through the waiting room, eyes cast down. Brian and Joan are waiting for me at the elevator, and when I see them, I break down all over again.

"We didn't get what we came for," I sob. They both hug me, and then physically support me as we leave.

Ten days later, I meet the specialist in a large, sunlit room. Lo and behold, a vase filled with tulips sits atop a gleaming white table, and Brian is able to select one of many chairs to sit on. The doctor is kind and doesn't try to talk us into the amnio; she says an element of risk exists either way. Instead, we choose to do a blood test and a thorough ultrasound, and this time we see the spine, the hands, the feet, and again our baby's heart beating healthy and strong. It's a girl.

We are elated. The specialist is pleased. She gives us the thumbs-up, and it's at that very moment that I begin to trust my intuition concerning everything to do with this daughter I carry. As she grows, so does a keen sense of knowing. Perhaps that's why I first chose Dr. R.—to push me to listen to that part of me that has always been wise.

—*Cheryl Montelle*

A version of "The Procedure" appears in the author's self-published book, My *Life and Paul McCartney: Collected Stories and Poems* (Motor Press, 2003).

Moments and Miracles

Four years and three surgeries ago, my husband and I figured it was time to add a second child to our family, since our firstborn was well past his first birthday. Many tears later, we have come to realize that the ability to have a baby isn't something that should be taken for granted.

We've endured tests, waiting room waits, and very personal questions. We've grieved the loss of a baby nestled into the wrong spot in my body. We've gone through adoption classes and home studies. Then, the unexpected happens. We are expecting.

"Finally!" is our son's comment when we tell him the news. In Timothy's elated anticipation of big brotherhood, he wakes Daddy at 3:00 A.M. to announce that he has thought of a name for the baby if it's a boy. He later comes up with a list of five suggestions, four of which honor the memory of his recently departed pet frogs.

When the time comes for me to be delivered from all the discomforts of pregnancy, I find myself on the couch in the middle of the night, timing contractions. I wait a little too long, as is my custom, and by the time I call the midwife to come and see whether it's time to go to the hospital, it is way past time. And it's too late to receive enough IV antibiotics to quickly knock down my strep infection, harmless to me but potentially fatal to the baby.

After a tense drive and an even tenser time gripping onto the admitting desk, my husband has to take off my clothes because I am in too much pain to do it myself. When the midwife checks me she announces in a surprised tone of voice, "You're ten centimeters!" I am not surprised. I am just happy to be in the hospital instead of the van. Things are not going as I'd envisioned them, quiet and calm, but rather fast and furious, and it is not long before I am yelling at the midwives, "Get it out!"

This is basically what they have been telling me to do, saying repeatedly that the baby has to come out on the next push because the heartbeat is dropping. This is easy for them to say.

"It's a boy!" someone says after what feels like far too long.

The baby is purple from having the cord wrapped around his neck, but vigorous enough to cry lustily. After some time, I begin to worry about his personality because he just won't settle. In the middle of the night, somebody comes in and tells us the baby's white blood cell count is abnormally high, and he needs to be treated immediately. They take him away.

I know a family that lost their perfectly healthy baby exactly this way. This is happening because I didn't get to the hospital quickly enough. This is all my fault.

The thought of losing him after all we've gone through is unbearable, unbelievable. My husband and I lie awake in the dark on separate hard beds, waiting and wondering. *Will we really have to say goodbye to him so soon after saying hello? Would God really take him away? How could our family go on if this baby dies?*

It seems an eternity before the pediatrician comes into the room, her white coat glowing like an angel. I ask where he is and if we can see him. They wheel me down to the nursery, and the sight of him—naked and startling under the bright lights, an IV line stuck into a tiny red foot—comforts me. He is alive and moving. He is real. I reach out to touch him and start to cry.

When the midwife comes in, she tells us not to worry, that the baby is in good hands. She means the doctors, but we know this statement has a deeper meaning. By the next day, the danger is already over, nothing short of a miracle.

Today I sit on a pillow on my computer chair trying to process what is behind and what is ahead. Daniel is twenty days old. He has prick marks on one tiny hand and both little heels. He has goopy, infected eyes. The whites of them are yellowed from jaundice. He has cradle cap, diaper rash, and bad baby acne. He has electrically shocked black hair and stork bites. He is absolutely beautiful.

When I hold this baby and think about what a miracle he is, I am awakened to the realization that every child is a miracle. Two microscopic cells meet and miraculously develop into ears, eyes, lungs, toes, a little nose, a pumping heart, a brain. A soul. One small body housing a whole new person—a special someone to love.

May I never forget these things. . . .

May I always remember what a treasure a child is. I am experienced enough to know there will be tough times. When he is teething or grumpy or stubborn or hyper, when he won't wear his mitts, when he pees his pants, when he draws on the walls, may I take a long view of things. When he forgets his homework and his manners, may I remember what I know today—that in the end everything will work out just fine. May I never be so focused on the demands of mothering a child that I am blind to the delights.

We have a lot ahead of us, this blue-sleepered bundle and me. I get to give him bubble baths and take him along wherever I go. I get to race cars with him, catch frogs, read adventure books, and play spy. Then I get to help him with his homework, and make him do his chores, and sit beside him while he learns to drive. I get to sob underneath my smiles when he stands at the front of a church, dark and handsome and wonderful, like his father on our wedding day. And then I get to let him go.

When this baby wakes for the third time tonight, may I savor the sweetness of his tiny fists on my breasts instead of worry about how tired I'll be. When he wants to play what seems to be the millionth game of Monopoly, may I not be blind to his smiles of togetherness. When he cracks up the car, may I be more thankful he isn't hurt than upset about the expense.

When it's all been said and done, may I have no regrets. May I not have missed the moments we walked through together on his journey to maturity. May I always remember that these are all moments to cherish, that my child is nothing short of a miracle.

—*Elizabeth Adam*

An Old Wives' Tale

It began during the third trimester of my third pregnancy. From a sound sleep, I would awaken with a raging fire rising from my chest to my throat. Unfailingly, the glowing numbers of the clock radio at my bedside would tell me that another night's sleep had been interrupted between the hours of 2:00 and 4:00 A.M. Even after the simplest, blandest of meals the day before, my nightly visitor would return: the heartburn from hell.

Having given birth to two daughters within the past four years, pregnancy-related challenges to the body were not unfamiliar to me. I expected nausea during the early months and figured I'd be home free once my first trimester was over. I could live with the other side effects—aching back, painful leg muscle cramps, frequent trips to the bathroom—but I was not at all prepared for indigestion of such volcanic proportions so late in the pregnancy. Perplexed, I consulted with my doctor during the next visit, who assured me heartburn was common during pregnancy, especially at night, when the mother-to-be was in a reclined position. He explained that it was caused by the growing fetus pressing against my stomach and recommended some of the milder over-the-counter antacids.

I bought and tried all three of the antacids, but each provided only temporary relief. The heartburn would go away for awhile but return an hour or two later, waking me up again. I read every pregnancy book I could get my hands on, hoping to find a remedy that actually worked. Dr. Spock advised more frequent and smaller meals and avoiding spicy and acidic foods. Another book suggested using an extra pillow to elevate the upper body. Still another recommended drinking a glass of milk before bed. No news there; I was already doing all of that, and none of it was doing a thing to relieve, much less prevent, the heartburn from hell.

"It means the baby is going to have a lot of hair," one of my friends told me when I brought up the subject at a play date with our children.

"What?" I snapped, wondering whether she was teasing me about something I didn't find the least bit amusing.

"Haven't you ever heard of that? It's an old wives' tale: If you experience a lot of heartburn while you're pregnant, the baby will be born with a lot of hair."

Frightening images of hairy infants swept through my mind—a tiny baby girl with hair piled high, à la Dolly Parton; a sweet baby boy with a mullet; a monkey-faced baby covered in hair, head to toe. I shuddered.

"That's ridiculous," I said "What could heartburn possibly have to do with how much hair my baby does or doesn't have?"

"I've heard it too," chimed in another well-meaning mom of twin boys, both bald at birth, if I remembered correctly.

"Well, I don't believe in old wives' tales," I said. "But if it's true, at this rate, we're going to need a barber on standby in the delivery room."

They laughed and then suggested the over-the-counter remedies they'd used while pregnant, each insisting that her antacid would do the trick. Neither of them did, not that I expected they would. By then, I was resigned to enduring the nightly heartburn for several more weeks.

One day in my eighth month, my mother stopped by and immediately noticed the dark shadows beneath my eyes. "You look tired, Maria. What's wrong?" she asked.

I told her of my problem.

"Vanilla ice cream," she stated confidently. "Try it when the heartburn wakes you up next time."

"Ice cream. Right," I said, too exhausted and irritable at that point to disguise the sarcasm in my voice. "Antacids don't work. Sleeping nearly upright doesn't work. Warm milk before bed doesn't work. But ice cream will? And why vanilla? Why not strawberry or chocolate chip mint?"

My concerned mother meant well, and she had more experience in these matters than I did. But she was, after all, the ice cream junkie in the family, and I couldn't help but doubt that plain ol' vanilla ice cream was the miracle remedy for my problem.

"It has to be vanilla," she insisted. "Just try it. It can't hurt, right?"

"I guess not. Anything to get some relief and some sleep," I answered.

Off I went to the grocery store while Mom played with my daughters. Turning up my nose in defiance at the medicinal aisle, I made a beeline for the frozen food section. I avoided the fattier brands and returned home with a carton of basic vanilla ice cream—the kind with those tiny flecks of vanilla bean—and skeptically awaited my experiment.

As expected, right around 2:00 A.M., the inferno within woke me up. I threw off the covers and quietly made my way downstairs to the kitchen, without waking up my husband or daughters. Removing a small bowl from the cupboard, I dished out one scoop. I sat down at the kitchen table and lifted the spoon to my lips. As each cool, soothing spoonful traveled downward, I could almost hear the upper portion of my body saying, "Ahhhhhhhh!" Instant gratification, if nothing else.

I returned to bed, tucked the pillow between my knees, and settled my big-bellied self under the covers once again. For now, anyway, the fire was out. I slept peacefully through the rest of the night. When I spoke to my mom the next morning, I told her that, while her sweet remedy may have worked this time, further testing would probably be necessary.

That night, while my family and the rest of the neighborhood slumbered in darkness, I returned to my kitchen at 2:30 A.M. and helped myself to another small bowl of the vanilla-speckled ice cream. Once again, the cold, creamy dessert extinguished the fire in my chest. I went back to bed, closed my eyes, and slept pain-free.

The same scenario took place every evening as my final weeks of pregnancy wore on. The heartburn intensified during the last month, but I kept my freezer well-stocked with vanilla ice cream. Night after night, a wonderful ice cream party-for-two would take place in the kitchen. Just baby and me.

Then, over Labor Day weekend, my reason for all that discomfort entered the world at 7 pounds, 3 ounces. He was placed in my arms, and I smiled when I saw his tiny head full of fine, dark hair. Once situated in the nursery, it was easy to spot him among the other newborns. The nurses had combed his substantial head of hair perfectly, with a part; he even had sideburns. We named him Christopher and brought him home a few days later. By the age of three months, he had his first haircut.

Now, at twenty-three years old, Chris makes regular visits to the barber on his own to keep his thick, shiny, dark hair neatly trimmed. Oh, and his favorite ice cream flavor throughout childhood and to this very day? Plain ol' vanilla.

—Maria Monto

Feeling Is Believing

I t's so hard to believe he won't get to see the baby,"
I sobbed into my husband's arms.

I was five months pregnant and had spent a
blissful summer day shopping for my first child's
nursery and layette, purchasing adorable furnish-
ings and sweet clothing that seemed impossibly
small. When I got home, I decided where to put
the crib and changing table and on which wall to
hang the yellow quilt adorned with pink giraffes
and blue elephants. Then I wrote passages in the
baby's memory book about the family members our
child would soon meet—and remembered the one
the baby would never meet. The next thing I knew
I was lying in bed, crying on my husband's chest as
he stroked my hair.

After five months of denial, it finally hit me that
my father, who had died nearly two years before, would

never know my child, and my child would never know him. Until then, I had been batting away the thought, swinging for the fence every time it came, of my father never knowing his first grandchild.

My father was my sole parent; I never really knew my mother. Her death when I was four left me with only two hazy memories of her. The sudden death of my father, when he was fifty-three and I was twenty-eight, was different. My dad had raised my brother and me alone, and he had been my dearest friend, always there when I needed him.

From the day I discovered I was pregnant, I had tried not to think much about raising children without him. It had been a struggle from the start. On the wintry afternoon that the home pregnancy test registered positive, my first impulse was to call my husband and then Dad with the happy news. Instead, after sharing the results with my elated husband, I called my brother.

"You're my second call," I said. "Are you ready to be an uncle?"

"Awwww, congratulations," he said, his voice cracking slightly.

A silence, filled with nothing and everything, passed between us. I hung up before either of us could cry and to meet my husband for a celebratory lunch.

Over the next four months, there had been plenty of distractions—morning sickness, business trips, buying our first home—to keep me busy and my mind off my dad's absence.

But as we prepared for our baby's arrival, I began thinking of Dad more frequently. Everything reminded me of him. I'd see an older man holding a little girl's hand or overhear a grandpa talking about his grandchild. Sometimes, I'd spot a bald man with a gray beard in a crowd and look twice to see if he was my father. I even had visions of my father with my child. I pictured him, with his thick hairy hands and Popeye forearms, holding my baby snugly to his chest. I envisioned him swinging my giggling toddler high above his shiny, clean-shaven head and then tickling a small, round cheek with his soft beard. I heard his deep, soothing voice beckon my pre-schooler from across the playground, promising ice cream after lunch and a ride home the long way, past the train yard.

By the day of the baby-things shopping spree, my will to deny that my father was gone forever had withered. Over the next two weeks, all I did was cry.

I finally called my brother, the only person who had known my father as I had.

"I can't get it out of my head that Dad will never see the baby," I said, perhaps still hoping he would tell me differently. "He'll never hold this baby or any other kids that you or I might ever have. How can that be, when he was our whole life?"

"I think he's watching," he said quietly. "I see him a lot, in my dreams. And I feel him, like he's near me."

I had not had that experience. "I believe he's with God, but I don't think he's watching me. I don't feel him like that. I think about him all the time, and I'm trying so hard to be open and believe that he's with me. But I just feel empty, like he's gone forever."

"Well, there is the due date," he reminded me. "Don't you think that means something?"

My baby was due on the very day Dad had died. "Yes, I do," I sighed. "I just wish I could feel him."

"He sees you now, and he'll see the baby, too," said my sage younger sibling. "Wait and see."

So I did. And he was right.

My son entered the world twenty-eight minutes after the day my father died. He was born with the same thick hands as his grandfather.

When my baby boy was eight months old, I dreamed of my father for the first time since he'd died. It was so real I could nearly feel his breath on my cheek as he said to me, "I see him. He's beautiful." I awoke in tears, grasping in the darkness for him.

Then, on the fifth anniversary of my father's death, my son, who would turn three the next day, broke a long and unusual silence as we were driving home from a sunny afternoon of play at the park.

In his precious little voice, he said, "Mom, do you miss your daddy tuz he died?"

I had not spoken of my father that day. I had never told my son of the date's significance.

"Yes, I do. Very much," I said, swallowing a lump in my throat.

He was quiet a moment before speaking again. "I'll be your friend now, Mom, tuz your daddy died. Otay?"

"Okay," I said, my voice raspy. "Thank you, honey." Looking up at the sky, I said it again, "Thank you."

—*Kimberly Charles Younkin*

Our Journey Back

Burke is the perfect image of his father, and he is the son we nearly didn't have. The year we were planning our fourth child, my husband, Dick, had a heart attack. Though it left no perceptible damage to my husband's heart, the pall it cast on our lives lingered long after his incision was healed and the artery had adapted to the stent.

At the time, my husband was a popular high school teacher and enjoyed his work very much. During his recovery, Dick was unable to do many of the things he enjoyed, and our busy household kept me occupied, requiring him to fend for himself often. He spent more and more time alone, not wanting to go many places, and he became increasingly more withdrawn. Dick also experienced anxiety attacks that mimicked the sensation of angina, resulting in many trips to the emergency room.

The instability of the situation completely unnerved me, and I was deeply troubled by my husband's growing emotional detachment from me and our three children. I did not want them to grow up without his active involvement in their lives, and I missed the closeness the two of us had always shared.

Though I still very much wanted another baby, prudence kept me from bringing up the subject. How dare I imagine bringing another child into the world when our future seemed so uncertain. My more immediate concern was trying to figure out how to heal the spirits and reinforce the bonds of our existing family. I decided that we needed to do something to get us out of our rut and moving forward again.

"Do you think we'll ever take the kids to Disneyland?" I asked Dick one night.

"Someday, I guess." Dick shrugged and didn't look up from the newspaper.

"We should go while they're still little, when they still believe," I said.

"Flights for five of us would be expensive," he said, reminding me that we'd have to travel at peak times when school was out.

"Why don't we drive?"

"That must be thirty hours of driving! Are you crazy?"

We do have all summer, I thought to myself, and

set to work convincing him that a road trip to Disneyland was just what we all needed.

Dick is nervous about flying at the best of times; when he drives, he feels in control and relaxed. Plus, a road trip would allow us to take our time and make an adventure out of it by camping in interesting spots along the way. At first, planning the trip was little more than a game, using maps and the Internet to plot our way over the Canadian border and through the Northwestern United States. The planning soon became a shared passion, as Dick and I researched campgrounds and tourist sites, and eventually we mustered the confidence to commit to the trip. In early March, we booked the first campsite reservation at Yosemite National Park.

In July, off we went on a fascinating 26-day, 10,000-kilometer journey. We drove from our home in Calgary through two provinces and four states, staying in nine different campgrounds along the way. The excitement of the first few days made me feel like a super mom—ready to face anything, anxious to show my children the world. When we reached Mount Rainer in Washington, however, I was somewhat disappointed; the cool climate was all too familiar. Dick and I huddled around the fire in layers of clothes and jackets.

"I thought the weather was warmer in the states," I whined.

"It'll get better the further we move south," he said. "Besides, look at the kids."

The three of them were "playing house" nearby, pretending to be bears and chatting to each other in creative little voices. They didn't use any toys in their game. Various levels of tree clusters created an apartment-style home, and each tree stump had a role to play: one was a sink, another a table; others served as beds. Our oldest daughter, Robyn, was doing most of the directing.

"Father Bear, please pick up some milk at the store," she commanded. "Baby Bear, you need to take a nap."

The other two happily complied.

"They are lost in their game," I marveled. "They don't even notice the weather, do they?"

"Imagination," Dick said, smiling as he poked at the fire. "It's good for the soul."

After the first week, we slowed our pace, taking time to enjoy the scenery as it changed from arid plains to lush forests. Dick and I grew closer to the children and to each other. We also took time for solitude, for thoughtful personal reflection; there were many life questions to sort through.

Of course, there were times when each of us got impatient and frustrated. Following a ten-hour day at Disneyland, I suggested we walk over to Main Street and stake out a spot to watch the parade.

"Oh, c'mon, the last thing we need is to sit on a sidewalk. Let's come back tomorrow; we're all exhausted," Dick said

I insisted. "The kids will love it. It'll be a perfect ending to a wonderful day."

I gathered our tired two-year-old, Abby, in my arms and struggled to find a place to sit on the edge of a planter as we waited for the parade to begin. Slowly, Dick was persuaded by the cheerful music and the friendly faces of the crowd to join in the spirit.

Leading Snow White's float were the Seven Dwarfs, waddling along the edges of the route. In wonder, Abby watched Grumpy approach for a hug. I'm sure it never crossed her mind that he was an actor in costume. To Abby, he was real.

When the princess float approached, all three kids were in awe. Characters they had seen in movies and storybooks were before them presented beautifully in makeup, hairstyles, and brilliant attire.

Abby's eyes sparkled as she said, "Daddy, isn't Ariel lovely?"

He smiled at her, and then leaned in to kiss my lips. "Thank you." There were tears in his eyes.

One day as we were leisurely making our way back home, Dick said, "I've been caught up in thinking, 'What would happen if I did this.' Now, I'm starting to wonder what will happen if I don't."

By summer's end, we were expecting our fourth child. When we announced the news to family and friends, I allowed myself to gush over how grateful I was to be carrying another baby and how blessed we felt. Given the events of the previous year, I embraced this pregnancy with even more zeal than I had the others. It was different.

I didn't wish away the days of discomfort. Rather, I cherished the middle-of-the-night sleepless moments as time to be alone with our newcomer. I patiently accepted the cramps and twinges of pain as signs that my body was making the necessary adjustments to accommodate the miracle developing inside me. Having learned firsthand the wisdom of "this too shall pass," I reminded myself that my tiny guest would not be visiting for very long.

The mood swings and absentmindedness that arose at the most inconvenient moments were a source of humor, rather than irritation, for Dick and me. One day he found the electric knife in the fridge.

My entire being—mentally, physically, emotionally, and spiritually—was completely engaged during the pregnancy. I was more attuned to what my body needed to fulfill its blessed purpose. When I felt tired, I allowed myself to bow out early from activities. I ate fresh foods and enjoyed meals for the right reasons, without regard for the scale or my figure. With fascination, I watched the stretch marks develop over my thighs and the spidery purple veins peek through the skin on my calves in later months. Sciatica, inflamed-nerve pain common during pregnancy, worsened as the months progressed, but I didn't waste time complaining. Instead, I attended yoga class and visited a massage therapist often, and Dick prepared cold packs for my back at night.

The most important difference in this pregnancy was that Dick and I could share it with our children. They were now old enough to appreciate what was happening, and we included them in every way we could. When Dick brought the three children to the ultrasound appointment, my protective son, Blake, came to my side in the darkened room.

"Are they going to get the baby out right now?" he whispered.

"No, honey, we have to wait for Baby to grow a bit more. Look at the screen. Can you see something moving?"

He nodded.

"Soon you'll be able to feel the baby's kicks too," I said.

Sure enough, by the sixth month, the baby's kicks were strong enough for the children to see and feel them on my tummy. The delight on their faces made my heart soar.

At thirty-six weeks, false labor took us to the hospital. When I returned home that night, Robyn showed me her diary: *Mommy went to the doctor today. The baby did not come out. On April 20th, the baby will come. Not today. My tooth came out today though.*

My own journal entries for this period are unlike those from my other three pregnancies. They are shorter, with fewer details, but they are richer in observation of my feelings. When I returned to them recently, I saw that I had been truly living in the present.

The morning of my scheduled cesarean, I drew a bath in the quiet house, to contemplate and savor the last moments of pregnancy. As I smoothed water over my ballooned belly, trying to memorize its shape, Abby toddled into the bathroom.

"Mommy, can I have bath too?" she asked.

"Of course, honey."

She lifted off her nightie and slipped into the bubbles.

"Today our new baby will be born," I reminded her.

Abby tilted her head and asked, "Mommy, how do you get the baby out?"

My stomach flipped as a vision of the operating room came to mind. It had been months since I'd given the birth itself much thought.

Swallowing hard, I glanced around the room and caught Dick smiling at us from the doorway. He winked, instantly calming my nerves.

"Abby, is the baby a boy or a girl?" he asked.

"It's a boy baby," she said. "He'll be a boy just like you, Daddy!"

"Yes, just like Daddy." I said.

I sent up a prayer of thanks that Abby and Blake and Robyn's Daddy—my husband, my partner for life—would be right at my side to help welcome our new baby, Burke, into the world.

—J. A. McDougall

The Great Rabbit Chase

Some pregnant women bloom gracefully during the nine months preceding the birth of their children. They wear regular, fitted clothes until the seventh month and never gain more than twenty pounds. Their tummies look like tiny, round cantaloupes. They often hear the phrase, "You look so adorable!"

Unfortunately, I am not one of those women.

As soon as I see the extra pink (or blue) line on the home pregnancy test, I make a beeline for the pantry. I reason that my growing baby needs every nutrient available, and the more I eat, the more likely I'll give her what she needs.

Consequently, I do not look "adorable" at any point during pregnancy. And during the last trimester, the words, "huge," "whale-like," and "titanic" pretty much describe me. My stomach sticks out so far that I regularly knock things off tables and countertops. Once, I even managed to spill a freshly poured mug of coffee on myself at a very important conference meeting by turning sideways too quickly. *Bump!* Coffee splattered across the table, carpet, and floor right in front of an editor I desperately wanted to impress.

Oh, well.

Recently, in my eighth month of pregnancy, I was once again feeling like a gigantic, waddling duck. While the kids visited Grandma, I paced alone in our quiet house, trying to decide whether to attack the computer and catch up on work or to dive into the pile of laundry that needed to be folded and sorted.

I headed for the computer.

My home "office" is really just a nook in a corner of our bedroom. The desk faces a large bay window overlooking the back pasture of our small farm. As I began to type, something white and moving outside caught my eye. A rabbit! And it wasn't just a wild rabbit. It was my seven-year-old daughter's pet bunny, which she'd named Frosting, because she said it reminded her of a vanilla-frosted cupcake.

Frosting was loose from his pen and on the run. So, I quickly realized, were the four other rabbits that shared the wood-and-wire hutch my husband had built. When I stepped out onto the back porch, I saw five furry hoppers bound off across the backyard in various directions. Upon closer inspection, I could see where they had dug a tunnel underneath the pen to make their happy escape.

Panic seized me.

I was feeling pretty hefty, with my fifty extra pounds of pregnancy weight sticking out in front of me. But I knew my daughter would be devastated if we lost her beloved pet rabbit. I determined right then and there that I would catch Frosting no matter what. I figured if I could get him near the door of the pen, he might run back inside on his own.

I lunged for the mad white hare, who, of course hopped quickly away from me. I decided to change tactics, hoping that maybe if I could catch the others first, Frosting might join. Besides Frosting, we had one black rabbit and three gray ones that also belonged in the pen. I ran all over the yard, huffing like an old locomotive. But they outran me, almost like it was a game. I wondered what my neighbors were thinking. They probably couldn't see what I was chasing and could only surmise that I'd lost my mind in my enormous last month of pregnancy and was running around the yard, hither and thither, perhaps to induce labor.

Yet, I kept imagining my little girl with tears in her eyes, knowing it was only a matter of time before the neighbors' two Irish Setters would be feasting on rabbit stew. So, I kept up the chase.

At one point, Frosting raced down a slope toward the side of our house. I lunged after him, and in my eagerness to catch the little white runaway, I slipped and fell, landing on my belly. The baby! I should have given up at that point. I felt the hot tears forming in my eyes. Now, I was worrying about my baby and my daughter's bunny. Still, I kept going.

By a stroke of luck, I caught one of the gray bunnies by running behind him until he entered the hutch. Slam! I closed the door. One down, four to go.

My main goal was to catch Frosting, who happily munched the green grass that filled our yard during March. I frowned, remembering how much work I needed to be doing inside our house. Should I give up the chase and just hope the dogs weren't interested in tasty little bunny snacks?

Nope. I had to keep going.

After a few more minutes of dragging my humongous belly around the yard and still only one rabbit returned to the hutch, I decided to call my husband at work. Maybe he could come home and help.

"Can't you catch them yourself?" he asked me, after I frantically described the scene.

"I can't! I've tried," I told him. "But I'm so huge, and I fell down once on my stomach, and now I'm worried about the baby. Can't you please come home?"

"You shouldn't be out chasing rabbits when you're eight months pregnant!"

"But we have to catch Frosting before the dogs get him." I begged, pleaded, and maybe even whined. Yes, of course I whined.

He agreed to come home to help me. So I took a breather on the back porch, rubbing my varicose veins and apologizing to the baby in my belly.

At last I heard the rumble of his car tires on our gravel driveway. He stepped around the side of the house and saw me standing in the backyard, surrounded by four dashing bunnies.

"I slipped down the hill," I explained, pointing to mud on the knee area of my jumbo-sized maternity jeans.

"Let me get my baseball cap," he said. "We can use it like a net and maybe round them up.

So for the next twenty minutes, we ran around the backyard, husband and large wife, trying to corral the rabbits. Slowly, one by one, we managed to get the other two gray and the black pets back into the hutch. But Frosting seemed to be enjoying his mischief. He munched grass until we got right up on him, then bounded away full speed like the Road Runner. Finally, we cornered him from two sides, and my husband waved his red ball cap toward the white furry animal. Frosting looked at both of us with black, shiny eyes that seemed to say, "Well, I guess it's time to go home." I yanked open the pen door, and my husband flapped the hat toward the little cotton-tail until he'd hopped back in.

The chase was over.

After all the excitement, I felt like I deserved a nap. Forget the computer and laundry! I propped up my aching feet, downed a Little Debbie Oatmeal Cream Pie (aren't those packed with nutrition?), patted my global belly, and settled into a much-deserved snooze. And dreamed I gave birth to a giant white rabbit.

—*Heather Lynn Ivester*

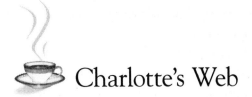# Charlotte's Web

I scoot closer to the edge of Miranda's couch as nausea, like the itsy-bitsy spider, climbs up my esophagus. My options are to make a beeline for the potted ficus or to navigate the minefield of toddlers at my feet to reach the bathroom. Pride and a fear that seeing me puking on "mommy's favorite tree" might leave scars on two-year-old minds, force me to choose the latter. I dart right to avoid a tea party, jog left to miss the music circle, and attempt a long jump over train tracks. Landing squarely on Thomas the Tank Engine is not at all pleasing to the arch of my foot, but it is even more distressing to Miranda's son, Liam, whom I hear sobbing as I dry heave over the toilet.

When the nausea subsides, I slump onto the cold tile, hold my head in my hands, and wonder how this pregnancy could be so vastly different from my first. During my pregnancy with Eliza, I basked in the miracle of developing earlobes and pinkie toes. I sang lullabies to my taut belly bulge so she would know the sound of my voice. I fear this baby thinks her mother is a drill sergeant, as I have been irritable and demanding since her conception.

I wipe away the tears and splash water on my face, hoping the moms will think the blotches are from surging hormones. As I enter the room, Eliza is announcing something to the group.

"Mommy doesn't like baby. It's a bad baby. It makes her sick."

I needn't have worried about blotches, as my face is now beet red with embarrassment. I sweep Eliza up under my arm, grab our backpack, and quickly thank Miranda for hosting. She tries to take my hand, but I brush it away saying, "I'm fine. I really think I'm coming around the bend with this vomiting. It can't last much longer. Thanks again! Bye!"

As I pull into the YMCA parking lot, Eliza's head falls forward like a drunk's. She's been sleeping in her car seat like this every day for two weeks, while construction workers tear apart our house and put it back together again. My guilt that she has to nap here rather than in her own bed is compounded by the fact that she's never complained, not about that or about having a grumpy mommy. I recline my seat all the way back so I can cry unabashedly, as six months of pregnancy misery washes over me.

The misery started during the second month, when my lungs began to rattle like the engine of an old work truck. The doctor diagnosed bronchitis and prescribed three hours a day of inhaling a steroid-free medication through a contraption of tubes and pumps called a nebulizer. With a Snow White figurine in one hand and an oxygen mask in the other, I'd attempt to keep Eliza entertained.

"Oh, you dwarfs did such a lovely job . . . (*Darth Vader–like inhale*) . . . cleaning the cottage . . . (*inhale*) . . . and I loved the whistling!"

When the gunk finally cleared out of my chest, my husband, Eric, decided it was a good time to replace the Pergo flooring with real wood. It would be a mess but, at worst, he assured me, a three-day affair. Two weeks later, and my kitchen appliances are still in the garage, dust covers every surface in my home, and the chemical smell from the finish is so strong I worry about its effects on Eliza and the baby.

So, here we sit in this parking lot, while workmen rip apart my home, plank by plank. But it is me that has come undone. I suddenly realize that this is too much for me to shoulder on my own. Pressing a button to raise the driver's seat, I rise like Frankenstein's monster and prepare to meet the unknown: asking for help.

As I stall on her doorstep, I see Miranda through the window. She is cleaning up the aftermath of the play date, a mess equivalent to thieves ransacking your home. Liam must be napping, which means I am interrupting her quiet time, the sacred hour or two that all mothers cherish. She glances out the window and spots me. My instinct is to duck out of view, but I give her a weak smile instead. Now, not only am I embarrassed about needing her support, but I'm also mortified that I appear to be a peeping Tom.

She answers the door with a bin of LEGOs in one hand and a tambourine in the other. Her face registers surprise that I have returned, but quickly changes to a look of knowing. She must recognize that I am close to a nervous breakdown.

"Let me guess; you need this," she says as she runs over to the coffee table.

What is she getting? Prozac? A suicide hotline number? A straight jacket?

"I thought this was yours," she says, shooting her arm toward me in triumph. She is holding a sippy cup. A flippin' sippy cup.

"Well, actually, no. I didn't come back for the cup. It's not the cup. It's that … I'm kind of losing it here, Miranda." And, once again, I break down in tears.

"Oh, my gosh. Come in. Tell me what's going on."

"I'm so sick and tired of feeling sick and tired," I say, slumping down on her couch.

I dump it all out, and Miranda listens in just the right way. No solving, no judging, just listening.

"Eliza is right, I'm not excited about this baby." I check for signs that Miranda thinks I'm a monster. Seeing nothing but compassion, I go on.

"Honestly, I'm so worn down I don't know how I'll get through labor and then take care of both Eliza and a newborn.

"But that's not even what I'm most freaked out about."

"What is?" she says, taking my hand in hers.

"What if I harbor some weird irrational grudge against this child for life?"

"You won't," she says.

I know she's right. But I'm surprised how good it feels to hear it—and to admit that I'm having a hard time.

"Would you like to bring Eliza in and put her on the guest bed?" Miranda offers.

I worry that it's too much of an imposition, but I'm so tired of the damn YMCA parking lot that I agree.

Miranda pulls back the covers for Eliza. With matted curls pasted on her forehead, my little girl looks peaceful. My sense of peace is being restored too. While Liam and Eliza nap, Miranda and I laugh, cry, and bitch, and it feeds my soul.

For the remaining three months of my pregnancy, I turn not only to Miranda but also to other friends who nourish me with compassion, understanding, humor, and best of all, occasional babysitting.

Then, a week before my due date, these friends gather at my house for a "blessing way"—a baby shower that focuses on giving the mother strength for the birth. Miranda comes early with dozens of candles. In the dim light, I can forget that the baseboard still isn't finished, and the room feels magical. As each friend comes in, balancing Tupperware containers and hot dishes covered in aluminum foil, we kiss on the cheek and exchange volumes wordlessly. My vulnerability fills the room, but in the presence of these women, it is strangely comfortable.

After sharing a delicious meal, we sit in a circle, and I am presented with a bead from each friend that I will thread into a necklace and wear during labor. I receive a gold bead shaped like a star—a gold star for enduring this pregnancy. Another bead is a swirling blue color, representing the ocean, reminding me to give into a current more powerful than myself. Another is a tiny bell whose ring signifies the little soul in my womb who will soon announce her arrival into the world. Once everyone has contributed, I balance the small basket of beads on my lap and run my fingers through each sentiment, absorbing my community.

Now, Suzanne, my birth coach, who has recently returned from Hawaii, performs a dance for us. I am mesmerized as she sways her hips to the Hawaiian music. She folds her arms as if rocking a baby who she tenderly kisses on the forehead.

Miranda reaches into her bag, pulls out a ball of red string, and instructs each woman to wrap a piece of it around her wrist. The result, a giant spider web connecting us all, makes us laugh. As Miranda cuts individuals free, she instructs them to tie the string and wear it until receiving word that I am going into labor. At that point, they will all cut their bracelets to signify the letting go that will allow me an easy delivery.

Two weeks later, my friends are still waiting.

"Any word yet?" they ask each other over the phone.

I am not surprised this baby is late. Why should she make things easy on me now? Ten days after my due date, Suzanne comes up with the idea of asking my friends to cut their bracelets.

"It will be a collective release. It will free you of the fear that is keeping this baby inside you," she says.

"Whatever," I secretly tell Eric.

Suzanne makes a phone call that trickles to everyone in the group. Within two hours, Eric is driving me to the hospital. Six hours later I am holding my sweet Charlotte in my arms. She is so beautiful and precious I laugh out loud at myself for thinking I could ever hold a grudge. That night, when we are alone in our hospital room, I tell her the miraculous story of how she introduced me to a village and how, with their help, she came peacefully into the world.

—*Emily Alexander Strong*

The Flowers in My Garden

I'm not a gardener. Without a miracle, I likely never will be. I have a black thumb. I'm convinced that if plants had feet, they would run screaming upon my approach.

For our first wedding anniversary, someone gave us a flowering indoor plant of some kind; I remember it was pink. At the same time, we acquired two kittens, who captured much more of my attention than the plant. The plant rapidly withered and died, and my astute sister noted that the kittens may not have much hope, either, under my care. But the kittens thrived, eventually becoming our "babies," along with a black Lab/German Shepherd puppy a few years later. They weren't quite the same as a real baby, though.

I am a baby freak. I love 'em—love the smell of milk on their breath, love their velvety little heads, love their petite toes with those impossibly tiny toenails, love those chubby rolls on their legs, love those sleepy sighs as they snuggle on my shoulder. As long as I can remember, I've wanted babies of my own. When Bryce and I married, we both said we wanted four kids. We never wavered from that.

Neither of us was prepared for the trouble it took to conceive. It was not an easy journey, and in the course of trying to deal with it, I tried many things to keep myself busy. Out of desperation, I even tried gardening. We lived in an 864-square-foot house in an old Portland neighborhood; I reasoned it could use a little outdoor sprucing. I failed miserably, and we ended up with weeds and a big patch of dirt in the yard. Next to our two neighbors—one who grew prize-winning roses and another who merely had to look at dirt to make flowers grow—our yard looked like a wasteland. It seemed like confirmation that I couldn't make anything grow.

At last, after two and a half years, we did conceive our first child through fertility drugs and an IUI (intrauterine insemination). Our son, Ben, was born ready to conquer the world. My best friend calls him a lion. He came out of the womb ready to take over—giving orders and expecting obedience.

I had no time to garden during Ben's first year. I remember being exhausted most of the time, but I also know I spent a lot of time savoring Ben's babyhood. I tickled him, kissed him, held him, slept with him—I treasured him. Being Ben's mom only confirmed that I wanted another baby. As he approached his first birthday, we decided to forego birth control again. We didn't know how long it might take to get pregnant again, and we didn't want to waste any time. Both of us were pleasantly amazed when I got pregnant right away.

Chloe arrived in early March, early spring in the Pacific Northwest. Her name comes from a Greek name meaning "new growth." She had long, dark hair from birth and big blue eyes framed by long, thick eyelashes.

Ben stayed with my parents until I was discharged from the hospital. Shortly after we arrived home, my parents drove up with Ben. My mother brought Ben up to the house with three daffodils wrapped in a wet napkin clutched in his chubby little hand. Mom always had daffodils.

Ben toddled over to the bassinet where Chloe slept and placed the flowers next to her head. "Here, baby," he said and patted her gently on the tummy.

"They were supposed to be for you," Mom whispered. "He was going to give them to Mommy."

From that moment, Chloe and Ben were rarely apart. As Chloe grew, she fought to keep up with Ben, refusing baby food in favor of finger foods and walking at eight months. Ben, being the good-natured, social kid he is, welcomed the attention. Through the turmoil of moving from a small, starter home into a larger, family home, Ben and Chloe were side by side, not entirely sure where one ended and the other began. I could hardly say one name without the other; through the haze of having two babies less than two years apart, they seemed joined in my mind.

The new home gave us elbow room. A quarter-acre lot and an extra couple of bedrooms and bathrooms made a huge difference to our growing family. We also had room to garden. Fruit trees lined the backyard, and the front was professionally landscaped.

"Maybe if it's started for me, I can keep it up," I remember saying.

Though I still wanted more babies, I needed time to breathe. With two children twenty months apart, me approaching my thirty-third birthday, and a new home needing some personal touches, I wasn't ready for another pregnancy. God had other plans for me, though; Chloe was eighteen months old when I found out I was expecting baby number three.

I remember crying as I told Bryce. I just didn't think I had enough hands to handle three children under the age of four. I worried the entire pregnancy, and it wasn't until about halfway through that I began to own it—began to accept and genuinely develop affection for the baby inside of me. Love was never a question; I knew I would love him. I just didn't know when.

Once again, gardening was put on the back burner.

Samuel was a wonderful surprise. Born in May, when much of Oregon is in full bloom, he was an easy baby from birth. Nine pounds, 6 ounces at birth, he rapidly gained enough weight to hold himself for a good sleep-stretch at night. By three weeks, he slept ten hours or more each night. At eight weeks, he laughed a full-hearted belly laugh—an indication of the influence he's since become in our family. By the time he was two, we could count on Sammy to make us laugh. He sings, he shows off, and he says silly things just to make his brother and sister smile. Ben and Chloe will argue with each other, but rarely with Sam.

The yard, however, has proven more difficult. By the time Sam turned one, I had pretty much given up on learning to garden. I began to picture a much lower-maintenance front yard—one with a brick patio that could be hosed off, maybe a few low shrubs that would need only an occasional pruning, and if—if—the urge struck, a small selection of annuals in the planter box. I thought that maybe the summer after Sam turned one, I might actually have some time to pursue a little yard work.

My plans for that summer came to a halt, however, when I discovered I was pregnant for the fourth time. I simply laughed. There was nothing else to do. From the beginning, I knew it would be the last time;

whether boy or girl, I would not have a fifth child. I braced myself for another twenty-month age difference and settled in for one last pregnancy.

It was a harder pregnancy than the other three. Though I had little morning sickness, I ached more, and exhaustion plagued me the entire nine months. At thirty-five, my body seemed to be telling me it was time to be done. I caught every illness that Ben, then in kindergarten, brought home, and at thirty-seven weeks, I ended up with bronchitis. I don't think I've ever been sicker. It just confirmed to me that my baby-making days had to end.

Natalie has not been an easy baby. She's serious, clingy, and shows early signs of being a shy child. She didn't sleep all night until about four and a half months old, even though I did everything the books say to do. But Natalie is a beautiful baby, and like her sister, she seems to be motor skills–oriented. I'm hoping for another early walker. When she smiles for me, it lights up her whole body, and I call it "my smile"—the one reserved only for me, the one not even Daddy can elicit. Because Natalie is my last, I find myself savoring the precious little things of babyhood even more than I did with her siblings.

After giving birth to four babies in six years, I think I can safely say that I know a little about pregnancy. My midwife told me with my last one that I probably could have just phoned in my vitals at each checkup.

My yard, however, is a mess. I know nothing more about gardening than I did back when we bought our first home. I have thistles, dandelions, and other weeds I can't even name running amok in the flowerbeds and grass. We did manage to get rid of some unruly grape-vines, and finances willing, will plant more flowers next year and put in that brick patio.

I'm not a gardener—never have been, and without a miracle, likely never will be. My children, however, are thriving. They are my garden. Ben is my azalea bush; he goes through dry periods when he seems not to grow at all, and then takes a spurt and flowers practically overnight. Chloe is a rose bush—a beau-tiful, tempting bloom with all the thorns charac-teristic of a second child, but also hardier than she appears. Sammy—darling Sammy—he's a daisy. He blooms with unabated optimism. He approaches the world with an open-faced, open-hearted enthusiasm. My precious Natalie, I suspect, is a tulip. I think she will lie dormant for a long time, and then cautiously peep through the soil, and then, when she is ready, bloom with blazing color, drawing people to her. I love every one of them and their unique beauty, gifts, and needs, and as a mother, I try to nurture those different needs to the best of my ability.

My babies are my garden. I envision lazy summer nights on that patio, watching my children ride their bikes in the cul-de-sac and chatting with the neighbors. With luck, I'll watch my adult children leave and come back home, again and again, to their roots. If I'm really blessed, someday my patio will be full of grandchildren, as lovely as any flowers, to admire.

—*Amy Rose Davis*

Waddling Down
the Strip

Jetting through the clouds over the Grand Canyon, Sam and I are on the way home from Las Vegas, our final fling before the baby is born. I'm six-and-a-half months pregnant, and we set up this vacation months ago, soon after learning we were expecting our first child. Besides having frequent flier miles that would soon expire, we were faced with giving up a freedom we've enjoyed together for years.

Fueling our own need to take this trip were other people's unexpected reactions to my blossoming condition, which have ranged from a waiter's caustic, "Well, get used to staying home," to a coworker's cynical, "That's sure going to change your lives forever." Even at the airport this afternoon, as a stressed mother carried her screaming child through the terminal, a complete stranger tapped my arm and said, "See what you've got to look forward to?"

I've tried to stay focused on the more positive comments, the ones extolling the joys of parenthood, but that hasn't prevented me from occasionally being gripped by fear as the due date rushes forward like a tidal wave. Usually, I am comfortable with our decision, but sometimes my confidence disappears like the shapely assistants of illusionist David Copperfield in one of the Vegas shows we saw.

My pregnancy was far from magical this past week. The day before we left for vacation, I became aware of a persistent dull pain in my lower back while I was at work. I nearly brushed off the symptom as one of those normal discomforts of pregnancy, but I didn't want to risk having a problem while we were in Vegas, so far from home. Because the phones in our office were temporarily out of service due to construction going on in the building, I went outside to ask whether I could use the phone in the construction site trailer. The foreman told me his phone was out, too, but drawled, "You ain't fixin' to have a baby, are you? Cause I can get you to a phone." After assuring him I was not in labor, I walked to the bank next door and asked the whereabouts of a pay phone. The loan officer took one look at my swollen stomach and, wide-eyed, handed me the receiver on her desk. I was advised to drive right over to the midwifery center and pee in a cup. As it turned out, I had a kidney infection and was given a prescription.

Between all the water I had to take with the medication and the baby using my bladder as a trampoline, I must have visited every bathroom in every casino on the strip. Each restroom, of course, had wall-to-wall mirrors, providing yet another constant reminder of my condition. I saw my pregnant self from every angle and also, for the first time, in motion. I now know I have a distinct waddle in my stride these days. There was even a mirror over the bed in our hotel room. Let me tell you, it is a scary thing when the first thing I see upon waking up is my very pregnant self waking up.

There were other reminders of my circumstance. I had to regularly apply sunscreen to my face, because I'm one of those brunettes who have the nasty side effect of chloasma or, as Sam affectionately calls it, "raccoon face." I also had a constant belly itch, resulting from a combination of stretching skin and dry desert heat, which no amount of cocoa butter could alleviate.

We did have a great time, though. Besides David Copperfield, we saw the Cirque du Soleil and took the scenic drive through Red Rock Canyon. We wandered through the medieval world of Excalibur, ambled through the lushness of the Mirage, and watched the talking statues in Caesars Palace.

On the last night, we were hot at the roulette table, and Sam convinced me to place all our winnings on a single last bet. It would be our grand finale, he told me. If we lost, we'd break even. Well, sort of. If the ball bounced our way, we'd walk away with a decent profit. Well, almost. With trembling fingers, I placed the stack of chips on red. Other players looked at us like we'd lost our minds, and I couldn't take offense at their accurate assessment. I was breathless as the little white ball spun around the wheel, defying gravity for a record-breaking length of time. It landed in black, bounced into green, and finally came to a wobbly stop in red. As I exhaled, Sam and I did a high five, then collected our cash and strode away winners. I choose to see that as symbolic.

Now, as we fly home to wash the stale smoke out of our clothes and prepare a room for the baby, I can close my eyes and see the roulette dealer waving his hand over the table and saying, "No more bets." We can no longer take back our wager. The stakes are high in this gamble of our lives. We have put our freedom and comfortable relationship on the line. The chips are down. But perhaps the payoff will be a life richer in love and a joy we can't even now imagine. We can only cross our fingers and hope as the wheel keeps turning.

—*April Burk*

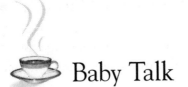 Baby Talk

I read some great novels while I was pregnant. I saw some good movies too. I might have even picked up some juicy gossip. But nobody gave a hoot. When you're pregnant, people lose all interest in discussing anything beyond your budding baby with you.

That might not be so bad if they offered useful advice. But the advice I got was about as useful as a string bikini after childbirth. My business-minded friends, for example, advised me to have the baby before the first of the year so my husband and I could deduct him on our taxes. Like I had a choice. Others were just as serious when they told me to wait until after the new year so the baby would get a free ticket to the Ringling Bros. circus. (The baby inherited my money-management skills and opted for the circus.)

Curiously enough, the most ridiculous advice always came from women who had children. One was a friend named Kathy. For a while, I imagined Kathy would be the friend I'd call every time I had a question about the baby. She had that laid-back, low-tech approach to motherhood that I wanted to emulate. When I told her I planned to breastfeed, she suggested I start brushing my nipples with a toothbrush to "toughen them up." Naturally, I added nipple-brushing to my shower routine. I would have kept it up until my delivery had the leader of my breastfeeding class not told me diplomatically that she'd never heard of anything so absurd.

Another mother with strange ideas was my sister-in-law's mom, Lenore. She told me that to raise a baby properly, I'd have to trade in my Civic for a van. After all, she reminded me, every time I took the baby out, I'd have to bring a stroller, a highchair, a playpen, bottles, a bottle sterilizer, a change of clothes for the baby in case he had an accident, a change of clothes for me in case the baby had an accident on me, etc. I didn't dare mention that my parents raised two reasonably well-adjusted children without ever driving anything bigger than a Chevy Impala; I was afraid she'd turn them in for child abuse.

Lenore's daughter, by the way, who didn't have children back then, told me very seriously that for as long as I was pregnant, I was not to lift my hands over my head. She must have expected me to keep wearing the T-shirt I had on for the entire nine months. She also told my husband that if it weren't for my pregnancy, she would have invited us for a ride in her boat. I suppose she was afraid I might lose my head and wave at a passing boater.

Of course not everybody I met advised. Some flattered. I don't know which was worse. The flatterers loved to tell me how lucky I was that I hadn't gained an ounce in my ankles. I guess they thought that would make me feel wonderful about the thirty-five pounds I gained everywhere else. My sister-in-law Lynn repeatedly told me that from the back, you couldn't even tell I was pregnant.

The folks I spent most of my waking hours with, the reporters in the newsroom where I worked, were refreshingly free of advice and backhanded compliments, if only because they didn't know a thing about pregnancy. But they did know about deadlines and seemed to resent the fact that I got away with repeatedly missing my delivery due date. On each of the ten days I was overdue, they'd give me that you-lazy-slacker look when I walked in every morning and ask why I wasn't giving birth. I tried to explain that a due date is not a deadline and that it's perfectly normal to be up to two weeks late. Then when I'd walk in the next morning, they'd start grilling me all over again on why in the world I wasn't busy giving birth.

While the reporters made me feel like I was dragging my feet, my friend Kitty made me wonder whether I was going to have a baby at all. Kitty was a great friend, for about eight months. I ate lunch with her several times a week, because she showed a genuine interest in me and not just my reproductive system. Then she started in with the Braxton Hicks. Braxton Hicks are contractions women have late in pregnancy. They're supposed to prepare our bodies for labor. As my due date neared, it became clear that my body was woefully unprepared. I would have preferred to keep this shortcoming to myself, but Kitty never gave me a chance. Every day she'd greet me with a big smile and a question about whether I'd had any Braxton Hicks yet.

Looking back on those nine months, it gives me great satisfaction to say that, unprepared as my body may have been, I made it through labor as well as Kitty had after her months of Braxton Hicks. And despite what the reporters thought was a pitifully late performance, I couldn't be more proud of the result. And I'm grateful I ignored Lenore's advice about getting a van. With gas prices hitting the roof, it's the reason we can still buy our son shoes.

So if you happen to get pregnant, take my advice and tell everyone that you're due at least a couple weeks past your actual due date. Save your toothbrush for your teeth. And if the going gets really tough, invest in a good set of earplugs.

—*Cynthia Washam*

Breaking the News to Grandma

The truth was there, and it didn't lie. As I watched the blue line magically appear on the white stick in my hand, my emotions went from hopeful apprehension to elation to anxiety in ten seconds flat. I was thrilled to be pregnant. What I wasn't so sure about was making the announcement to my mother: "Prepare for a grandbaby. Again."

I should have been elated to share the news. Happily married for nearly four years, my husband and I were perfectly ready to become parents. We had done "all the right things" in exactly the right order: high school, college, career; dating, engagement, marriage; save money, buy a house, get a dog; have a baby. After all, I was the responsible middle daughter, the one Mom seldom had to worry about. She would be tickled to hear I was pregnant, right?

Yet, my palms were sweaty as I contemplated what should have been the happiest day of my life. Would she embrace my news? Or would she see it as just another responsibility?

My predictable life had been overshadowed by other demands facing her. Mom became a grandparent at age forty, when most women are still raising children. In fact, her children were still children when my two sisters, each barely out of high school, blessed her with a grandson and two granddaughters. For them, motherhood hadn't been a picture-perfect beginning.

One of my sisters was eighteen, unmarried, and struggling to make ends meet when she announced her big news to Mom. My other sister was living out of state with an abusive husband when she announced she was expecting twins. She also revealed that he had hit her once in the stomach after learning she was pregnant. An unwed mother-to-be? An abused, expectant mother? How earth-shaking was my announcement next to those?

My sisters had needed our mother emotionally and financially during and after their pregnancies. One sister walked away from her abusive marriage and moved in with my parents when she was six months pregnant. With no husband in the picture, she needed Mom to hold her hand in the delivery room and to give her a hand in caring for the baby.

The other sister was forced to leave her newborn in Mom's care and travel overseas on a six-month military assignment. When one sister struggled with drug addiction, Mom invited her kids over for weekend stays that turned into week-long and month-long visits.

As I nervously stared at the white stick in my hand, I realized I could never compete with my sisters' needs. Mine was too simple. I just needed my mother to be happy about my pregnancy.

After a visit to the doctor confirmed the home pregnancy test results, I tried to think of a simple way to tell my mother that she was going to be a grandparent again. I decided to wait several weeks, until Mother's Day, to break the news. I purchased two greeting cards for her. The first featured a standard Mother's Day greeting; inside, I wrote a simple note of appreciation and love, and signed my name. The second card was much smaller and featured a Mother's Day greeting for a grandmother. On this one I wrote: *You are going to be a grandmother.* I slid each card in its respective envelope, and then placed the smaller envelope inside the larger one and mailed it off to my mother.

After several days went by with no response, I left a message on my parents' answering machine, asking if they had received the card. Another day went by; still no response. I wondered whether the cards had been lost in the mail or whether she had somehow missed the smaller card. I wondered whether she'd been too busy, perhaps with the grandchildren, to open her mail. I waited and wondered. Finally, on Mother's Day weekend, I received a phone call from her.

"I got your card," she said. "That was nice of you."

I waited for her to say something else, like, "Oh, how sweet of you to tell me your news on Mother's Day," or "Why didn't you tell me sooner?"

Her matter-of-fact tone and brevity of words left me stunned. Was she really not happy for me? I was hurt by her aloofness and contemplated saying something like, "So, I'm on my own with this pregnancy? Too much for you to handle?"

Her next response surprised me.

"I haven't opened the card yet. Your dad got the mail a few days ago when your card came, but he left it in the car and just now brought it in."

"Well," I said a little too quickly. "Have you opened the card?"

My mother must have detected the urgency in my voice, because I immediately heard the sound of paper being ripped open and the card being pulled out.

She read the card out loud to me: "'Thank you for being such a good mom all these years. I appreciate you. Love, Shanna.' . . . Well, isn't that nice. Oh, and you've included a gift certificate."

The suspense was killing me. "Go on," I urged. "Open it up."

Again, I heard the sound of paper rustling. Then, she read the words aloud, and I thought I detected a slight catch in her voice when she said "grandmother."

My mother—already well-practiced at being her daughters' maternity support system, delivery-room coach, and much-needed second mother to their children—let out a soft sigh. I could only imagine what she was thinking as I waited for her to say something, anything.

"Oh, Shanna," she said. "Congratulations."

It was spoken in the warmest, sweetest voice I could have hoped for. The truth was there, in the tone of my mother's voice. And it didn't lie. Mom was happy for me. She seemed happy for herself, too . . . maybe even tickled about being my baby's Grandma.

—*Shanna Bartlett Groves*

A version of this story was first published as "Reluctant to Be Pregnant" in the self-published book, *150 Ways to Creatively Announce Your Pregnancy* (Booklocker, 2005), edited by Heidi Gonzales.

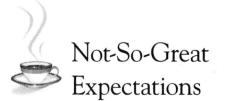

Not-So-Great Expectations

The chanting could have been my imagination, considering I was in my third trimester and looking it. I was enjoying the sunny day with a stroll through the park when it started. Just a whisper at first, it grew louder as I walked. I admit that I was proud I finally looked pregnant instead of chunky, and maybe my outfit was a bit on the snug side. It's possible I did strut past the two old men sprawled on the park bench, but only because I was thrilled with being a mommy-to-be. Besides, surely they'd seen pregnant women before.

As I walked away from them they called out in a loud, bawdy, sing-song chant: "We know what you did, we know what you did." Nope, it wasn't my imagination. I knew it was probably just the alcohol in the brown bag they shared talking, but that didn't stop the heat from rising to my face. I wasn't embarrassed.

Not really. Sex is a completely natural act, and what I did with my husband behind closed doors was none of their concern. It was what they'd reduced it to that got my pulse pumping.

Trying to convince myself that my flushed cheeks and racing heart were the result of the crazy hormones surging through me, I decided I'd walked enough. Pretending to ignore the raucous laughter trailing behind me, I climbed into my car and flipped on the radio. Spilling out of the speakers was one of those commercials, with a sad little-kid voice that turns your heart inside out. Even as I realized my mistake, I knew it was too late. Already, tears streamed down my face, and I was so mesmerized by the sweet voice that I couldn't change the station. After searching in vain for the tissues I'd forgotten again, I gave up and used the back of my sleeve to mop at my face. That could have accounted for my failure to see the concerned policeman until he tapped on my window. When I explained that I was fine, that it was just a pregnancy thing, he leaned over, casually placed his forearms on the window opening, and proceeded to tell me, in detail, about his wife's emotional roller-coaster through her three pregnancies.

Ten minutes later, my composure finally regained, I pulled out of the parking lot. I'd gone nearly a block when it hit me: I was starving. How could I be so hungry when I'd eaten only an hour ago? But I

absolutely knew that I had to find a box of Fig New-
tons, so I bypassed the convenience store and headed
to Safeway. Deciding that, since I was already there, I
might as well stock up on other stuff, I grabbed a cart.
I hadn't made it down the first aisle when I saw her—
a tall, beefy woman on a mission, heading straight for
me. She raced down the aisle, expertly blocking my
cart to prevent escape, determination etched on her
face, wicked enjoyment gleaming in her eyes. I knew
what was coming: childbirth horror tale number one-
thousand-eight-hundred-ninety-three.

When I was newly pregnant, I'd envisioned
myself as part of a special sisterhood of women who'd
been there, done that. I'd imagined other mothers
extolling on the virtues of pregnancy and little old
ladies patting my tummy with fond memories of
their own reproductive days. Apparently, I'd ended
up in the wrong sisterhood—one called "Bad News
Mamas." In the ensuing weeks I'd heard it all: nausea,
vomiting, unexpected bowel movements, leg cramps,
backaches, swollen feet, puffy faces, breech births,
C-sections, cords wrapped around necks, late births,
early births, days of agonizing labor, making it to the
hospital with thirty seconds to spare, not making it
to the hospital at all. I even heard about a baby who
fell out while the mom washed dishes at the kitchen
sink. Why did so many women insist on telling me
how awful pregnancy and childbirth were?

I couldn't do it. I just couldn't force myself to listen to another stranger's nightmare. So, when my polite "excuse me" didn't deter the cart-blocking woman at Safeway, I took the only option left. "I really have to pee," I called out in a panicked voice, abandoning my cart as I raced out of the store as quickly as my waddle would allow.

Realizing that no grocery store was safe anymore, I headed to my oldest sister's house. For one thing, Judy is the one who'd taught me that fail-safe method of escape, and I wanted to thank her. Plus, I wanted to raid her fridge. As I fed my ravenous belly, I updated her on my morning adventures. It must have been a combination of my hunger and hysteria and her concerned silence that made me careless. Before I could stop myself, I was asking for advice. What was reality? What was myth?

Now, under normal circumstances, I know that the four people on this earth I can count on to tell me the truth, whether good or bad, are my four sisters. They give it to me straight and don't hold any punches, knowing I'll be stuck with them anyway.

Judy was the first of us to have a child. In her no-nonsense way, she instructed me to ignore Mom's description of what the delivery would be like—a virtual walk in the park.

"Mom told me that contractions are like bad menstrual cramps," Judy said. "They aren't. I still haven't decided whether I'm going to forgive her for that."

I knew my sister could hold a grudge, but since this one is pushing seventeen years, I started to worry.

Judy also informed me that my Lamaze teacher would try to convince me that it's not pain I'll feel during labor, just pressure. When I asked if that was the way it had been for her, she gave me a smile and patted my hand. "Yes. Labor can be called pressure, just like a tornado can be called an air current."

When she started in on the list of creative names to call my husband, explaining I'd appreciate having them handy during the delivery, I decided it was time to go.

Looking for distraction and maybe a bit of com-passion, I called Karen, my second oldest sister. She met me at my house with a surprise—"the box," she called it, holding it out like a family heirloom. Thinking it would be full of fun baby things that would make me cry but would be well worth it, I dived in. I'd barely made it through the top layer when I knew I had the wrong box. Why would she bring me two packs of super-duty menstrual pads, complete with safety pins? And what was that pack of huge old-lady panties for?

When she explained, I did cry, and it wasn't because of the cute baby things buried in the bottom.

Why hadn't anyone told me that the menstrual cycles I'd happily missed during my pregnancy were simply hiding and gaining power, like a tidal wave, and would rise up and swamp me once the baby was born? And I was planning a vaginal birth, not a C-section, so why would I need those extra large panties with room for bandages?

"Just in case," she said.

I escorted her out the door, shut and locked it behind her, and proceeded to pace the floor. After a day of drunken old bums leering at me in the park, a crazed woman trapping me with her grocery cart at Safeway, and my very own sisters scaring the bejeebers out of me, I was rattled. What had I gotten myself into? Could I handle it?

Giving in to my anxiety, I called Mom. I wasn't about to ask any questions about what my body would go through before, during, and after the delivery. My sisters had covered all that well enough. I needed to regroup, to remind myself why I had done this. I decided to focus on my baby, what she'd be like. My latest pregnancy book assured me that the best way to get this information was from Mom.

As soon as she answered the phone, my questions spilled out. How much did I weigh when I was born? How long was I? Did I have hair? What color? She listened patiently without comment, letting me unload. Given that she'd had eight of us (I have three brothers too), my mother's response should not have surprised me.

She summed it up in two sentences. "I remember the first and the last. The rest are just a blur."

Great. I'm number seven.

"Mom," I complained, "How is that supposed to help me figure out what my baby will be like?"

"Okay," she relented with a chuckle. "I may not remember the details, but I can tell you that you were all average, between six and eight pounds. You all had hair, but since you're one of the blonde ones, yours was so light and fine you might as well have been bald."

Running my fingers through my shoulder-length hair, I thanked her and hung up. Knowing it was time to face my fears of the upcoming event, I started flipping through the packet of information from my doctor's office. Putting aside the information on Lamaze, I found the schedule for regular childbirth classes, the ones for women who believed in epidurals. It didn't say that exactly, but since it was included as an option under "pain management," I figured it was as close as I'd get.

With my husband's screwball schedule, the only class we could attend together was a single weekend course named "Prepare, Plan, Park, and Push." I wondered if they'd purposely omitted the word "panic" from the title. Registration took fifteen minutes, and most of that was an overview of my personal information. When was I due? Not soon enough. Was this my first? Yes, or I wouldn't need a class. Was I planning on having the baby at the hospital? I really, really hoped so. I was just finishing the registration (and was already exhausted) when my husband walked in and gave me an amused look. I slammed down the phone and struggled to my feet. How dare he be amused? After the day I'd had! Ready to explode, I considered storming after him but was stopped by the image of myself waddling like a pathetic duck. Instead, I slammed my hand on the counter to get his attention.

He turned, wearing a grin so wide it probably made his cheeks hurt. In his hands was a pair of Winnie the Pooh booties with little rattles on top. I simply melted. The tears came again, this time out of relief and joy. As we talked about the little girl who would soon be joining us, the frustrations of the day slipped away.

The next morning I woke up with a solution to the trials of the day before. Rather proud of myself, I got to work and had just finished when my husband came into the kitchen.

"What's this?" he asked, picking up the sheet of paper with a cord attached to two ends.

"I'm going to wear it when I walk in the park," I explained, "to get people to leave me alone."

"'I'm not pregnant. I'm just fat,'" he read. He flipped it over to read the other side. "'Yes, I'm scared. Satisfied?'"

"How about this instead?" he asked, scribbling on a blank piece of paper and holding it up for me to read: *Pregnant and proud of it.*

"You don't understand—," I began.

"What I understand," he said, kissing me on the cheek, "is that you're carrying our baby, our miracle. Don't you think it's natural for people to be drawn to that, to want to be a part of it?"

Conceding it was possible, I placed his sign on the passenger seat. Maybe I'd wear it, maybe I wouldn't. Just in case, my sign was tucked underneath.

—Wendy M. Campbell

The Mother of All Jobs

Carrying the last of my personal belongings, I walk to the door of my classroom, leaving behind a completed substitute plan, the only sign of my presence remaining in the room. I take one final look around before locking the door for the last time and making the solitary walk to my car, the last one left in the parking lot. I let the tears fall as I drive away, not knowing for sure when or whether I will return. I am proud of my job and that I can name my place in society. I am a teacher. *Who do I become tomorrow when I don't open the door to my classroom and greet my students as they walk in the door?* I wonder. I am more scared of losing this sense of who I am, even if it's only for a semester, than I am of anything else in my life.

I realize that this is still true the following morning when I am awakened by a tickling on the inside of my leg. I look at the clock; it is 5:00 A.M. If this is my husband's idea of an invitation for intimacy, he has made a big mistake. With a ridiculous amount of effort, I heave my body onto my left side to glare at him, only to find him fast asleep. *Hmmm.* Slowly, the cause of this unfamiliar sensation dawns on me. My bag of waters has broken. *This is it,* I realize, with a slight sense of panic. *I am going to become a mother.*

"Who are you? How would you describe yourself?" the magazine article I read the night before asked. Last night, the answer was easy. I am a high school teacher. I love my job. I like adventure. I am a good listener. I am . . . pregnant. The last statement didn't pop into my mind as easily as the others had, and even though my belly has grown to the size of a mansion for my child-to-be, it is still hard for me to incorporate this fact into my identity. I am going to be a mother. It won't be long until I will also add this word to the list of traits that describe who I am. It will definitely take some getting used to. The mere thought of this word, "mother," brings to mind an unfortunate image of a frazzled woman with uncombed hair, bags hanging under her eyes from too little sleep, a shirt that doesn't match the pants because the one that does is covered with baby spit-up. My nausea returns. I don't want to become this woman. I can't become this woman. I feel claustrophobic knowing that at forty weeks and three days into this pregnancy, at this point, there is no other way out. I plead with myself not to become this woman, but if I don't become her, then who will I be?

With the impending onset of motherhood and all the joys that it is supposed to bring, I am panicked by my feelings of loss, both of myself as an individual and of my place in society. I have just handed a job I love over to another teacher so that I can go out on maternity leave. Although I had always cheerfully thought that I would stay home with my kids to nurture them and help them grow, now that the time is here, I don't know if I can really do it. *What if I whither away or slowly go mad at home? What if I am overcome with guilt if I decide to return to work? Is there any "right" decision?* I ask myself in between contractions on the thirty-minute drive to the hospital.

My husband glances over worriedly each time he hears my breathing change to cope with the surges in my body. He sees the look on my face.

"Are you scared?" he asks.

"About the birth? No, not really."

He doesn't catch on that I am very afraid, just not for the reasons he thinks. It is not the labor or the pain or the impending delivery that worries me. I trust my body. Women have been giving birth for thousands of years. Our bodies know how to do this seemingly impossible task. He doesn't probe any deeper. He never finds out that while I trust my body to give birth I don't know whether I can trust myself to know how to mother. Or to want to mother. That I'm worried I won't be able to provide for someone so small and so dependent. That in a matter of hours I may lose myself completely.

Four hours later, after one final push, my baby makes his way into the world. I am exhausted. I have given all that I have to give him life and I have nothing left. His slippery purple body is placed on my only slightly smaller belly, and without any conscious effort, I feel my arms instinctively curl around him, providing both protection and warmth. I open my eyes and stare at him in wonder. He stares right back. The cutting of the umbilical cord marks the final separation of his body from mine. We are now mother and son. We are no longer one. We are, I realize, individuals.

Two weeks later, feeling guilt-free, my husband leaves the house for his first day back at work. I am left alone with our son and a decision to make: to return to work in a classroom for pay or to work at home for . . . for what? For the chance to change diapers and be spit up on? No, I realize, looking at my son. It is for the chance to be there to see the first smile and the first step, for the chance to raise a member of the next generation. Wiping my son's urine off the bathroom mirror (don't ask), I realize that, for the first time, the answer is clear. Although the job of a stay-at-home mom is rarely glamorous, the hours are brutal, and the monetary compensation is terrible, this may be the most important job in the world. The rewards of this job come not in the form of bonuses and raises but in a baby's smile and the pleasure of narrowly avoiding a stream of urine. Though I know that as a stay-at-home mom I'll never be named employee of the month or teacher of the year, I will forever see the lasting results of a job well done. It is a tough and selfless job, but somebody has to do it and that somebody is going to be me.

Even though I sometimes feel as though I've lost a part of myself now that I don't work outside the home, I have gained a greater understanding of who I really am. I am still a good listener. I still like adventure. Though my class size has dropped to one precious student and my classroom has expanded to become the world in which he lives, I am still a teacher. Above and beyond all that, I am a mother. I work harder than I have ever worked in my life. I enjoy and am proud of what I do. And I am pleased that, for the moment, I am not covered in spit-up.

—*Amy Booth*

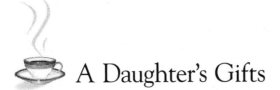

A Daughter's Gifts

My mother and I stood on the front porch as my father loaded the last of their luggage into the car. They had a two-day drive ahead of them, from my home in New York to theirs in Michigan. My daughter, Ella, just seven days new, yawned while I held her in my arms. That first week of Ella's life, my mother had showed me how to change her, bathe her, dress her, hold her, nurse her, and most important, how to comfort her. Mom was a calming force during a chaotic time of round-the-clock feedings and recovering from the delivery. She also cooked meals and cleaned my house.

Mom gently cupped Ella's tiny face in her hands and kissed her on the forehead, and then she hugged me. "It's a very special thing to be a mom," she said as she pulled away. Her eyes watered, and a small smile played across her lips. "Welcome to the sisterhood."

I watched my parents drive away, feeling lost and utterly alone.

For many years I prided myself on my independence. Being the oldest of four kids, I was expected to help my mom take care of my younger siblings. I resisted and resented this responsibility as only a teenager could. They didn't like it any better, and they responded with, "I don't have to listen to you! You're not my mom," and slammed doors.

"Why should I have to watch these little brats?" I'd lash out at Mom.

"Why can't you help me? You always have to be so difficult," she'd snap back at me.

On and on, the angry words flowed back and forth between us.

As I grew older, the chasm between my mother and me grew wider. Not only did we have very different views about my responsibilities to my siblings, we also had vastly different personalities. My mother has a larger-than-life persona. A flashy extrovert, she could start up a conversation with anyone, while I preferred keeping a more low-key, behind-the-scenes existence. We were worlds apart, and I couldn't wait to be out on my own.

After college I moved away, far away. I focused on my career, and my mother started telling people I was not interested in having children. Whether she had gleaned this from comments that I had actually made or from how I dealt with the sibling-sitting, I'm not sure. Communication between the two of us was sporadic and strained at best. By then, I was convinced that mothers and daughters just did not get along well with each other.

During my mid-thirties, I met the man of my dreams and got married, and before long we were pregnant. Panic set in. How would my mother react? The baby would be her third grandchild, so my apprehension wasn't because she was uncomfortable with the idea of being a grandmother. She seemed to dote on my siblings' children. What worried me is that it was my child. Will she be excited or think "ho hum?" Will our relationship taint her feelings toward my baby? Even more pressing were my own reservations: How do I feel about having a child? Especially a girl child? I cringed at the thought of another turbulent mother/daughter relationship like the one I grew up with.

To my vast relief, both of my parents were thrilled when they heard about their newest grandchild. They immediately planned the trip to New York so that they could be there when my daughter and I came home from the hospital.

While they were visiting, I saw a side to my mother I don't remember ever seeing before. There was tenderness when she held my daughter. Mom cradled Ella in her arms like a precious package and spoke to her in quiet, soothing tones.

My mother sat with me while I nursed my daughter. She entertained me with tales of my brothers, sister, and me growing up. I had heard most of the stories before, but they took on new meaning for me now. One story in particular made an impression on me.

My family moved when my sister, the youngest, was six weeks old. Mom told me how she was nursing my sister after just moving into the new house when my three-year-old brother got his head stuck in the metal railing on the stairway. That's when the Welcome Wagon woman showed up unexpectedly and wouldn't leave. I began to realize the extent of the frazzled state she continually lived in with four kids. My father worked long hours and much of the time she took care of us by herself.

The week came to an end. My father had to return to work. When they left, I thought I would be alone. We had moved to New York a few months before the birth of our daughter for my husband's job and knew few people there. Because he was new at his job, my husband worked long hours and couldn't take off much time.

After my mother got back to Michigan, she began calling me every few days. I'd give her an update on the baby's progress—her first smile, how much she had grown, when she first rolled over—and then I'd ask my mother questions.

"What was it like when . . . ?"

"Did you have this problem . . . ?"

I found myself asking her more and more questions. We'd chat and compare notes. As I began to understand what she had gone through as a mom, the rough edges of our relationship, and my heart, seemed to smooth. Eventually, I found myself picking up the phone just to talk to her and to fill her in on the latest Ella stories. Somewhere in those string of phone calls, Mom started to say, "I love you," at the end of the call, and I found myself responding with a quick, "I love you, too." The phrase that once barbed my tongue now came naturally.

The first time my mother saw Ella, she commented, "Nice nail beds." I pictured them in the future going to get their nails painted—yet another interest my mother and I don't share, but the image made me smile.

I am sure there will be stormy times ahead for Ella and me, but I have faith in change, in mothers and daughters, and in the power of new life. Having a child has been a gift in more ways than I ever imagined. It gave me a daughter and healed the bond with my mother.

—*Laura Schroll*

A Friend in Deed

I have always been lucky with my neighbors. As first-time homeowners, my husband and I had a retired couple on one side of us and a young couple with two toddlers on the other. The older couple offered valuable advice on raising roses, the other on raising kids. At our next house, we were equally fortunate to enjoy lovely mid-summer chats over the fence, sharing gardening and barbecuing tips with neighbors on all sides. We've had snow-shoveling neighbors, babysitting neighbors, and a handyman neighbor. Then there was Carole. She was full of life, full of heart, and full of opinions. Things were never dull when Carole stepped in the door.

Of course, at that point, life was never dull for me, anyway. After years of being unable to have children, we fell suddenly into parenthood with the arrival of our beautiful adopted daughter. Soon after, we moved with our new baby from a big city to a small town. Life changed dramatically, and we rode the waves of good times and bad, navigating our way through the challenges of raising a bundle of energy who demonstrated daily that she had a mind of her own.

Sometimes I felt overwhelmed with the daunting task of parenting a spirited child and wondered whether I was up to the job. After years of longing to have children, to experience the miracle of pregnancy and childbirth, I was now almost grateful that the possibility of my conceiving a child was remote. As much as I adored my daughter, raising her seemed to take every ounce of energy, creativity, and sanity I had in me. *One is enough*, I told myself.

Carole lived a few doors down the street, and we quickly became friends. Her husband was a pilot and was often away for extended periods. My husband had a demanding job that kept him late at work, often well into the evening. Carole and I joined forces, sharing suppers, playtimes, babysitting. I'm not sure how much she benefited from my support, but I know I couldn't have survived without hers.

We walked our kids all over town and took them to the park, tiring them out so they would go to bed early and sleep soundly. My daughter was on the verge of giving up afternoon naps, a depressing thought for me, since I craved that hour or so of relief when I could read or write or just sit without having to respond to anyone else's needs.

In the summer, we lounged on the edge of Carole's backyard pool, sipping pop or tea and watching our little fishes at play. We talked about everything from world issues to the latest gossip in town while our children spent all that frenzied energy in the water. It was fun and relaxing, and I know it was good for our children.

By the time my daughter was five, I was looking forward to the next fall, when she would enter school full time. I had relished being a stay-at-home mom, but now it was time to get back out into the world and to scratch my creative itch. I taught a night course in English as a second language to adults. The local community college was looking for someone to teach children's literature, which happened to be my specialty, as well as someone to teach a business communications course for small business owners the next year. Having my daughter in full-day kindergarten would free up the daytime hours for me to pursue these teaching positions and for my own writing. It was all falling into place.

In early April, I started to feel unwell, not all the time, only at moments during the day. At first I thought nothing of it. *Just tired,* I assured myself. *Just not eating right.* The idea that I might be pregnant never occurred to me. How could I be? We'd been told it couldn't happen, that it would never happen.

The home pregnancy test said otherwise.

My husband was thrilled, and so was I—but I was also in shock. A new baby meant putting all my plans—of returning to fulfilling work outside the home, of having time and solitude to write, of improving our family finances, of being a positive role model for my daughter—on hold.

Then there was the age factor. A first pregnancy at forty is not a simple matter. Although I knew I was fit and healthy and physically younger than most women my age, I still lay awake at night praying the eternal prayer of mothers-to-be everywhere: *Please let my baby be all right.*

We didn't tell anyone at first, deciding to get the first trimester safely behind us before announcing our news to the world.

Carole came for supper one spring evening, tired after a day of caring for her nephew, but ebullient and chatty as usual.

"Thank goodness my kids are older now," she said. "I'm exhausted after a day with him. He's a good baby, too, so it's not that he's any trouble. But, oh, the diapers, and having to watch him constantly, and picking him up and putting him down, and heating up bottles—!" She sagged into her chair at my kitchen table, where we were sitting with our tea after supper. The kids had moved outside to play before evening fell. We could hear her son and daughter chattering as they ran and my daughter laughing trying to keep up.

"Aren't you glad you have only one?" Carole asked, shaking her head as if to clear it. "I love my two of course, but another one? No way—"

"Carole—" I tried to interrupt, but there was no stopping her once she gets rolling.

"—I mean, who'd want to go back to baby land? All that work—"

"Carole—"

"—and no sleep—"

"Carole—"

"—Sure, they're cute and all, but—"

"Carole—"

She stopped and looked over at me. By now I was crying, tears rolling down my cheeks and plopping onto the cooling surface of my tea.

"Oh . . . " she breathed, her mouth round with surprise. She didn't say another word, because she knew immediately, without me telling her, as soon as she'd taken note of the untouched food on my plate, the paleness of my face, and the tears that flowed without stopping.

Carole reached over and took my hand—and for the next seven months she held it, literally and otherwise. She walked beside me, a steadying presence for this forty-something mother facing her first pregnancy, anxious and uncertain.

When my son was born, it was Carole who showed up first to see him. She sat at my kitchen table and held him gently in her arms. "Oh, you're so lucky," she whispered to me, smiling down into my baby's sweet face.

—Jean Mills

Disassembling Momma Hen

I am not particularly fond of covering my kitchen walls and counters and linens with cows and ducks and other cute barnyard creatures. There are other quirky things going on there that probably shouldn't be construed as decorating. But it's the best I can do.

There is, for example, my mother's rolling pin. Why she owned one, I don't really know, because she couldn't bake. For that matter, neither can I and I don't intend to learn anytime soon. I keep it because it keeps my husband on his toes, like it kept my father on his. You just never know what the women in our family are capable of.

There is also my great-grandmother's splintering, long-handled wooden spoon. It is my magic wand, and everything it stirs tastes like gourmet heaven. There is a small, simple crate with a tattered label on it that pictures fading but still juicy peaches. I will never replace it, no matter how disintegrated it gets, because the nickname of my oldest child is the same as that fruit.

A cheap plastic plate hangs in a place of honor. On it is the scrawling, simple artwork of my baby, now a grown man. It sports a too-round woman's face, smiling, with bugged-out eyes. It looks too much like me for comfort. Beneath it, in a crayoned child's hand, it reads: Mommmy. With three m's. I'll never part with that, either, even when the artist starts sprouting grey hairs in his chiseled, manly beard.

There is one more eclectic thing in my kitchen: a milk-glass covered dish. The lid is a hen, and she is opalescent white everywhere, except for a bright red beak. The dish part is the same pearly white and covered with fine-tooled faux rickrack basketry. The piece is one of those items that is best kept carefully cherished and dusted and safely away from children. Except it never has been.

When I was little, I used to sneak up on it when my own mother wasn't looking and carefully—oh so carefully—lift the mother hen up to peer inside. Deep within its dish sat a real, tiny nest. It was tightly woven from delicate twigs, as if the hen had spent days crafting it. As a child, I had no way of knowing that the glassworks hired basket artisans to weave such magic.

Now, I don't know why that nest held such fascination to me. Maybe it was because it was so perfect and small. Maybe it was because the first time I'd found it, it was an unexpected surprise, like something really good at the bottom of a Cracker Jack box. But time after time, I found myself drawn to it. After looking all around, back and forth, to make sure the coast was clear, I'd gingerly pluck the little nest from the mother hen and cradle it, giving it a good look over.

My mother caught me one of those times, which was bound to happen.

"What are you doing?" she asked, as she wiped her hands on her apron. (They were still wearing them then.)

"I don't know."

The sight of me looking up sheepishly with an empty nest in my hands was too much for my mother to bear. She laughed almost until she cried.

"I do," she said, taking my secret treasure and placing it back inside the momma hen. "It's because, sometimes, even when you know something is there—but it's hidden and you can't see it right away—it doesn't seem real. But there it is, isn't it?"

Huh? The gravity and wisdom of my mother's words were lost on me then. I was just happy I hadn't been sent to my room. It would be years before I understood what she'd meant.

Momma hen became mine after my mother died. It was the first thing I set out in my bachelorette kitchen, a couple of blocks from the beach. There was sand everywhere in that place, and I sudsed momma hen gently every couple of weeks to keep her gleaming white. I always took a few moments to hold her nest; my mother would have expected that.

I married, and the kids started coming. Momma hen watched them grow from her perch in my kitchen, where she sat and fairly clucked approval the day my son came home with my portrait on a plate. He and I were hanging it on the wall for the first time when I heard a clunk.

My daughter, then about the age I'd been when my mother found me out, was standing with the nest in her hands and the top of momma hen at her feet. She began to cry. My palms began to sweat.

"You okay?" I asked, wiping my hands on my jeans, not owning an apron. I confiscated the nest and checked her hands for cuts.

"Uh-huh." She nodded and sniffled.

Momma hen looked intact, and I set her back in place over her nest.

"By the way—what were you doing?" I asked.

"I dunno."

In a sudden case of déjà vu, I found myself speaking in my mother's tongue: "It's because, some-times, even when you know something is there—but it's hidden and you can't see it right away—it doesn't seem real. But there it is, isn't it?"

My son shook his head and wandered out of the kitchen. My daughter nodded lamely, and I knew what she was thinking: *Whatever. I'm just glad I didn't get in trouble.*

Many sunrises have risen and set in my little kitchen. My daughter stopped disassembling momma hen a long time ago, and began collecting college credits and boyfriends and eventually wedding gown fabric samples. Not long ago, she and I were sitting in my kitchen and chatting, while I downed coffee and she patted her growing belly, full of my second grandchild.

Her firstborn—my granddaughter—was with us, and she lay an ear on her mother's bump. Hearing nothing, she shrugged and got busy with her dolls on the floor.

My daughter got up, waddled over to the counter and picked up momma hen, brought her to the table, and called my granddaughter over. She is a well-behaved child, not like me or her mother, and hadn't yet found out the secret of the hen. My daughter lifted the lid, and my granddaughter's eyes grew bigger and bigger when she saw the little nest. From my daughter came the same words spoken by me and my mother before me. And as soon as the words had left her mouth, she looked at me and we both laughed.

Recognition (and not the sullen confusion of her mother and grandmother) flashed across my granddaughter's face. Turning again to her mother's swollen figure, with the most serious tone she addressed her sibling-to-be: "Hey, you! It's time to stop hiding in there!"

Momma hen may be a quirky family heirloom, but she is also the tie that binds our womenfolk together. She is the keeper of the mystery of life, a reminder that we hold within us the gift of life. And so, from generation to generation, we pass the nest.

—*Candy Killion*

Mother's Intuition

I hit my shoulder against the interior of the car door as I rushed to open it and tumbled out, barely staying on my feet. The smugglers I had been chasing had already crashed their truck into the ravine and fled on foot, and I had narrowly escaped dumping my patrol car into the same ravine. Another car with flashing lights and a screeching siren skidded to a stop in a cloud of dust behind me, and another state law enforcement officer leapt out of his truck with a shotgun. "Which way?" He yelled at me.

I pointed off to the east as I started running in that direction. A helicopter was already swooping over the area, and I adjusted my radio as I ran. The voice of the spotter on the helicopter crackled into my earpiece. "We've got them. They're hiding in a wash, under a tree. You're heading in the right direction."

This was part of my life as a rural law enforcement officer. I loved this life, even though it really is 90 percent boredom, 9 percent complete frustration, and 1 percent pure terror. One moment I was helping a stranded motorist change a tire on a rural highway, the next I was pursuing drug smugglers off a dirt road and plowing through the desert where there was no road. Now, I found myself running through the scraggly bushes and the hot sand, gun cradled in my arms, eyes peeled for any one of the bad guys to pop their heads up and take a potshot at me. The situation required absolute concentration . . . and I was not concentrating.

My feet pounded on the sand and my lungs burned as I ran, but I hardly noticed. An image of my little brown-haired second grader unexpectedly danced in front of my eyes. She was what I liked to think of as my "breaking-in baby." She was my firstborn. She was the one I worried over, for whom I boiled everything she touched, and about whom I called the doctor and her grandma for advice all the time. She was the one born purple with the cord around her neck, but who rebounded with gusto, growing strong and healthy and smart. She was the one who looked just like the old pictures of her daddy, my husband.

I still worried about every little thing as she grew. She knew it, too. "Don't worry, Mom. I want to go to school," she told me solemnly on the first day of kindergarten.

I shifted the gun in my sweaty hands and changed my course slightly in response to the helicopter's instructions. I could hear the other officers, two of them now, pounding along on either side of me, spread out so as not to present an easy, tempting target. In my mind's eye, I also saw my younger daughter, my little blond toddler.

We called her our "special projects baby." She was born with two congenital conditions. One necessitated regular visits to a pediatric cardiologist, who assured us that everything would be fine, one day, either naturally or by surgery. The other condition meant that at seven months old, she had abdominal surgery to remove a life-threatening cyst. I saw my husband the way he had been that day, standing in the hallway of the pediatric prep unit, cradling her in his arms, tears in his eyes. My big, burly ex-Marine, clutching that little bundle to his chest, while two doctors and three nurses pleaded quietly with him to give her up.

"It's time for us to take her to surgery now, sir." The anesthesiologist said, trying the gentle authoritative approach. My husband didn't even look at her.

One of the nurses said, "You have to give her up now."

He shook his head.

Another nurse laid her hand gently on his arm. "We have to take her now." Again, he shook his head. She added, "You'll get her back."

His wet eyes focused on her, and she seized on it as a sign. "You can see her as soon as it's over." She put her hands on our baby, and he loosened his grip a little bit.

The anesthesiologist said, "We'll take good care of her."

The nurse and doctor tugged a little bit together, and he let her go. We stood watching as they carried her down the hall. She stared at us with her big blue eyes but never made a sound as strangers bore her off through the double doors. They closed behind her, and she didn't see her daddy collapse in tears.

I thought of my children's father, my husband of more than ten years. Job stress, family stress, and life stress had taken its toll on our marriage, and it was only in the past year or so that we had gotten the counseling and help we needed to fix what was broken between us. It was like getting married all over again, to a new man, who was also the same man who had sat those countless nights in the children's hospital, dosed fevers, kissed ouchies, and made it home every evening after I left for work to make dinner, bathe the kids, and put them to bed. He even did dishes.

It was not unusual for me to think of my family while I was on duty—off and on, while cruising in my patrol car on a calm night or after helping a family in crisis. But not incessantly. Not with such intensity. Not when I was in a situation that required my full attention. Lately, it seemed like everything reminded me of my children.

The voice of the helicopter spotter buzzed in my ear again. "You're almost there; bear a little bit more to the right. You should be almost in sight of them. They aren't moving."

As I closed in on their position, I should have been thinking of what I was doing. Instead, I was thinking: *What am I doing? If I get killed in the next few minutes over a few hundred thousand dollars in drugs, will that matter to my kids when their mom is gone? If I leave this job, will they even miss me in a few months? Someone will take my place, and I will have been no more than a ripple in the water to them. But if my kids lose their mom, it will change their lives forever.*

We closed in on the suspects, yelling instructions in English and Spanish. With my partners holding guns on them, I crawled under the bush and handcuffed the men and removed any weapons they had. One by one, they squirmed out from under the bush. We had apprehended them without violence. This time.

But something inside me had shifted. Suddenly, this career that I had dreamed of and worked so hard for had lost its appeal. The job hadn't changed; I had. I knew deep down and without a doubt that it was time to stop.

Within a month, I resigned my position and left the department. My husband said we would manage without my income somehow. If I felt that quitting was the right thing to do, then it was the right thing to do, no matter the cost.

Three days after my last day of work, my little one asked, "Mommy, aren't you going to work?"

"No, honey," I said. "Mommy doesn't work there anymore."

"Why not?" she asked.

"Because," I said and paused a moment to think. Why not, indeed? I'd loved my job and yet I'd quit my job.

"Because, honey," I said, "you and your sister are more important. Because being your mom is the best job ever. Because this is where I'm supposed to be, here with you and your sister and—"

That's when it hit me. In that instant, I knew what I should have known all along, what my mother's intuition had been trying so desperately to tell me. There was another reason why I needed to change my life before I messed up my most important job, as the mother of my three children: It turns out that on the day I decided to end my career as a law enforcement officer, I was already pregnant with my "new life" baby. I had joined the department to make a difference in people's lives, but I finally realized the place for me to make a difference was at home. I had been speeding through life too fast to see what was passing by, and it took the screeching tires of renewed motherhood to get me to pull over. Trade my badge for dirty diapers? Sure. I had a whole different kind of road to patrol now, with a lot of similarities: graveyard shifts, accidents, candy "smugglers," and dangerous behaviors to catch and prevent. I have never looked back, never regretted that decision. Not once.

—Nancy Clements

I'm Having What?

Triplets. That's what one of the ultrasound technicians was whispering to the other. At six weeks, it had been twins. Now, at eight weeks, it was triplets? Thoughts raced through my head. *Three is great. Three is fine. I can do three. Please, God, don't let it be four.*

I suppose three at one time sounds like a lot to most people; it certainly did to my husband. I gave him the good news in the hallway by the elevators and then laughed as he tried his best not to faint. He was scared, I was thrilled, and neither one of us was prepared for what was about to happen. This pregnancy would be nothing like those our friends had experienced, nothing like the ones we'd read about.

We'd started trying two years before. I was thirty-one, healthy, and hopeful that a month or two of wild, wonderful sex with the man I loved would see us on our way to becoming parents. We had everything planned out: a three-bedroom starter home, a station wagon, a little money set aside. Our baby would be born in late spring, and my husband, a college professor, would have the whole summer to bond with our child before classes started again in the fall. That was the plan, anyway, but that one month stretched into twelve, despite a small fortune spent in ovulation predictor kits and pregnancy tests. Thirty-one and hopeful became thirty-two and desperate.

The infertility testing started about the time I'd expected to be discovering the joys of motherhood. Instead of counting tiny fingers and toes, I counted progesterone suppositories. Life wasn't working out the way it was supposed to. I had a college degree and a successful career; what I really wanted was a baby. My cousins, who had put family ahead of work, were spectacularly successful at having kids. Loads of kids. Beautiful babies and ringleted toddlers. Apparently, somebody had their priorities all wrong. Family gatherings were torture until my priorities and my ovaries straightened themselves out.

When I rushed to the bathroom that first morning, we thought something was wrong. How ironic that after two years of trying to have a baby, we didn't recognize morning sickness when it hit. It's true, though, we didn't even think of trying the pregnancy testing kit we had hidden away under the bathroom sink. We went straight to the doctor's office.

Things progressed smoothly for a while, even though pregnancy was not at all what I had expected. I never threw up after that first day, though I gagged every time I brushed my teeth. I never had any food cravings, not even for pickles and ice cream, but I did have food aversions. One, in particular was so severe that I threw away not just the food but the bowl it was in as well. Still, I got big fast. Just four months along, I was as big as most women are at full term. And walking hurt; it always felt like one of the babies was trying to fall out.

All things considered, however, I felt great. For the first time in my life, I had boobs! And even if my belly was huge, my fanny wasn't, and I looked pretty darn good in those black spandex maternity pants. But all good things must pass, and when I woke up one night to find blood running down my leg, I thought my pregnancy was over.

It was one o'clock in the morning, the Monday after Thanksgiving, just eight hours before my scheduled five-month checkup. My husband helped me to the car, and I lay down in the front seat, not crying yet, but absolutely certain I was losing the babies. We didn't talk the whole way to the hospital.

There was a pregnant couple ahead of us at the sign-in desk. The desk clerk, who'd obviously seen it all before, told us and the other couple not to worry; she'd be with us in a minute. She meant no harm, I knew, but I couldn't afford to be patient or polite.

"I'm five months pregnant with triplets, and I'm bleeding!"

I think it was the snarl on my face as much as what I said that got the clerk's attention. Immediately, she hustled me into a wheelchair and sent me off to a room, where my husband and I waited, terrified of what the morning might bring.

It brought answers (just a polyp) and surprises (preterm labor). I would not be going home any time soon. They moved me from the observation room (a cold, pink hell where *Happy Days* was always on the television) to a bright, sunny room with soft, white blankets, a recliner for my husband, a TV/VCR with a remote control that I could reach, and my very own refrigerator—almost heaven.

The first month I felt like I'd won a free vacation to a part of the world I didn't necessarily want to see. The view wasn't great and neither was the food, but it beat the heck out of working. I spent my days and nights in bed, eating, reading, and watching television. A T-pump taped to my leg delivered a drug that postponed my delivery. The telephone and occasional visits by my former coworkers staved off some, if not all, of the boredom. And although I hated the idea of spending Christmas in the hospital, I knew my babies' lives depended on it.

While the world outside prepared for the holidays, my husband brought Christmas to me. He decorated a small tree, strung lights around the room, hung tinsel on my hospital bed, and joked about how we'd better enjoy our presents this year because next year we'd be spending all our money on the babies. Life was good. Then, a few days before Christmas, the T-pump stopped working.

I celebrated Christmas that year in grand, albeit unusual, style. Instead of the traditional glass of eggnog, I toasted my friends with a round of magnesium sulfate (that stuff will bring a glow to your cheeks, let me tell you). Instead of Christmas carols, I hearkened to the electronic beeps of my babies' carefully monitored heartbeats. Instead of sugarplums, I settled into morphine-inspired dreams of rats, Darth Vader, and a mountain of tangerines. Finally, instead of opening presents, I had my cervix sewn shut. The only thing I remember about Christmas day itself is the gift I gave to my parents: the names of their unborn grandchildren.

Things grew more intense as my belly got bigger: sponge baths, iron shots, painful IVs of white goo that looked and felt like the frosting on my thirty-third birthday cake, 6:00 A.M. cervical checks, and more rounds of magnesium sulfate. I swelled to 167 pounds—almost as wide as I was tall. I felt like Violet Beauregarde (the blueberry girl) in *Charlie and the Chocolate Factory*. Only thirty weeks into my pregnancy, I couldn't imagine how I would feel if I made it to the prescribed thirty-six weeks.

As it turned out, I didn't have to. My babies were born by cesarean section at thirty weeks and six days. Maggie, my black-haired beauty, was first. Robbie, as fair as his sister was dark, came second. Pete, with flaming red hair and a temper to match, was third. My husband and I saw them for brief seconds before they were whisked off to the neonatal intensive care unit where they would spend the next month.

That was six years ago. Today, Maggie, Robbie, and Pete are healthy, strong, and smart. Looking at them now, you'd never know that they almost didn't make it.

Strangers smile when they see the triplets. "You had your family all at once," they say.

I nod and grin, mindful as always, that it nearly wasn't so. Nothing about that pregnancy was what I expected it would be, but bringing home my babies was more than I ever dreamed.

—*Terri Reagin Gibson*

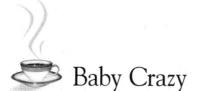

Baby Crazy

When my fifth child was born, I grieved a little, knowing that Owen would more than likely be my last baby. My rational side argued that five beautiful, healthy children were enough—more than enough, according to a few of my friends who affectionately christened me "crazy" for wanting a house full of kids. As I packed away my maternity clothes, I recalled, with some amusement, how much I had changed in thirteen years. Somehow, I had been transformed from an astonished and terrified woman facing impending motherhood to a contented and happy mom, pining for just one more baby.

I was the baby in my family and one of the youngest children in the neighborhood. Babies were scarce while I was growing up, and in any case they held little interest or appeal for me. While the other little girls played with their dolls, fine-tuning their maternal instincts, I spent my childhood capturing bugs and begging my older brother to let me join him and his friends in their adventures. When the woman next door brought her new baby home from the hospital, I was pleased by the prospect of increasing my income with more babysitting jobs, but I honestly couldn't see why everyone was making such a fuss over the rather ordinary-looking, red-faced bundle.

I grew to love my neighbor's new baby, but caring for her didn't inspire me with dreams of having my own children. I graduated from university and began teaching first grade. I enjoyed working with young children, but I wasn't sure it was something I wanted to do for the rest of my life. I contemplated returning to school to become a veterinarian—something I had always dreamed of doing. However, plagued by uncertainty once again, I chose to remain in teaching. Then, I married my longtime boyfriend and before long we bought a house, but still, I was restless. I tried to ignore the nagging sense of feeling incomplete. Something was missing. I was happy, but not contented. I was accomplished, but not fulfilled.

My husband and I both wanted children, but nothing definite had been decided. When we were both twenty-nine, I became pregnant. Everyone was thrilled, including me—on the outside, that is. When I thought no one was looking, I slipped into a private fog of doubt and more than a little anxiety.

I found myself overwhelmed by the growing realization that I was now entirely responsible for another human being. No brain surgeon facing a lifesaving operation felt any less accountable.

My self-confidence fell to an all-time low. *Do I have what it takes to be a good mother?* I wondered. *Can I do it?* When I finally voiced my doubts to my mother, her eyes told me I had nothing to worry about, and her smile told me she loved me for wondering and wanting to know. Then she reminded me of a night years before when I had been looking after the newborn baby next door.

"Do you remember the time you phoned me because Lizzie wouldn't stop crying? You were terribly upset, so I went over to see if I could give you a hand."

I nodded. "Of course, I remember. I felt horrible. Nothing I tried seemed to help."

"She had a touch of colic, poor little thing. But when I walked in, you were sitting on the living room floor, rocking her and talking to her—having a conversation with this screaming baby, in your calm and quiet voice, and rocking her the whole time. And then she stopped for a moment."

"She was just catching her breath," I said.

My mother laughed. "Probably, but she did stop, and when she looked up at you, I remember thinking that Lizzie knew she was loved and that someone cared."

"Really?"

"Yes, really. And you did it all on your own. You made the baby feel that way." She gave me a hug. "You're going to be a terrific mother."

A month after my son, Gabriel, was born, I didn't feel very terrific. Just before the baby's arrival, my husband had accepted a job that took us 600 miles away from my family, and I had yet to make any close friends. Gabriel woke up two and sometimes three times a night, and I stumbled through my days in a sleep-deprived stupor, feeling far more like a fraud and a failure than the terrific parent my mother had predicted I would be. When he cried—something he did with what I considered to be alarming frequency—and I tried to comfort him, he would squirm and struggle as though he didn't want to be held. Worse than any feelings I might have had was the thought that I was letting my baby down.

Our family doctor reassured me that Gabriel was a normal, healthy baby and suggested that I join a mothers' group that met each week. As much as I wanted to meet new people, I couldn't picture myself telling anyone that I felt like a terrible mother and, worse yet, that I didn't think my baby liked me.

Then one night when Gabriel was about six weeks old, I woke up with a start at about 2:00 A.M. Time for a feeding, I thought, and swung my legs over the side of the bed. Suddenly, I froze, paralyzed by the unfamiliar silence. Gabriel wasn't crying. Something must be terribly wrong. My heart pounding, I hurried down the hall into his room. When I realized he was okay, I rested my head on the edge of the crib and closed my eyes for a moment. When I opened them again, he was staring right at me and, as I watched in amazement, a smile appeared on his little face. When I picked him up, he relaxed in my arms, as if to say, *I'm feeling a lot better about this whole situation. How about you?*

The sleepless nights were far from over, and I still suffered from the occasional lapse in confidence, but the message of that moment stayed with me, loud and clear. Being a new mom was no picnic, but neither was being born. Some babies—just like some moms—needed more time to get used to things.

I joined the mothers' club and made friends, but the biggest changes in my life came from within. I found myself waking up with a sense of wonder and anticipation more frequently. Most nights I went to bed looking forward to the next day—something I hadn't done for a very long time. It occurred to me that I had stopped thinking about what I wanted to do with my life.

Just after Gabriel's second birthday, I became pregnant with my second child. When I found out that my son would soon have a brother or sister, I was elated. It wasn't just the thought of a new baby that delighted me. I was thrilled by the prospect of another pregnancy. My bewildered friends recounted their horror stories of morning sickness that plagued them twenty-four hours a day, of swollen feet and swollen hands, and of the betrayal of their bladders and their bodies. Of course, they gladly endured these discomforts and inconveniences, because, after all, their trials had been rewarded with a most precious gift. But pregnancy itself? "No thanks," one of my friends said with a smile. "Just give me the baby."

But then you'd miss it, I wanted to say. They'd miss what I still consider to be among the most remarkable moments of my life—the incomparable experience of creating life and giving birth, of being partner to a miracle. I endured my share of pregnancy woes—the nausea, the exhaustion, the never-ending hormonal rollercoaster ride. The sight of a supermodel flaunting her flat stomach could reduce me to tears, especially combined with the vision of my ever-expanding rear end. *That can't possibly be me,* I'd think, peering over my shoulder into a mirror.

I comforted myself with the knowledge that it was all temporary. Before I knew it, the new baby would be here. Watching Gabriel dress himself and ride his tricycle—when it seemed like only yesterday that he was a baby in my arms—confirmed my suspicion that somehow time was going faster than it ever had before. Gone were the feelings of emptiness and the moments of wondering, *What should I be doing?*

Emily arrived a week early, slipping into our lives as though she'd always been there. When Dylan was born two years later, his place was waiting, too. Three babies, all different, but each remarkable in his or her own way and each giving me a sense of purpose—and joy—that I never knew existed before they entered my life. When I became pregnant with my fourth child, Connor, my Aunt Helen, a mother of six grown children, teased me that I had inherited the "addicted to babies" gene from her. The birth of my fifth child, Owen, when I was forty-three, provided further evidence that she may have been onto something. But I wasn't just addicted to babies; I was in love with the whole package. As my children grew from babies to toddlers and from preschoolers to teens, I found new reasons to rejoice in being a part of their lives.

I still experience fatigue and frustration. There are times when I crave a quiet space of my own and question my sanity, but those moments pale and lose their significance when I think back to the days when I wondered what to do with my life. Now I can't imagine doing anything else.

—*Susan B. Townsend*

Doctors Are a Mom's Best Friend

I stumbled into the bathroom Saturday morning and thought my weeklong flu was going to win. I'd never felt this sick in my life.

"Honey, why don't you go see the doctor?"

My husband held my hair back while I lost the contents of my stomach for the umpteenth time that day.

I shrugged. "It'll pass. I'll be fine soon."

I sipped the diet ginger ale he offered a few minutes later. Was this the flu? Or something worse? I'm a diabetic, and serious infections can send my blood sugar haywire, which means a trip to the doctor. But I don't like doctors. So I didn't go … until my five-day flu extended its stay to two weeks and showed no signs of leaving. I couldn't avoid it any longer. Something was wrong. I went to the doctor's office, where they poked, prodded, and did a full blood workup.

Did I mention I'm not fond of doctors?

A few days later, my husband met me at the door as I was returning from work and told me the doctor's office had called. He had some news, and I should sit down.

"Honey . . ." He took a deep breath.

This must be one nasty infection, I thought.

"Honey . . ." Another deep breath.

Oh, no. It's worse. I have some incurable disease.

"Honey, we're going to have a baby. You're pregnant!"

I sat utterly still, in stunned silence.

Switching gears from sick beds to baby beds took more than my brain cells could handle.

"Are you okay?" he asked.

I opened my mouth to answer but didn't know what to say. No? Yes? Maybe? I was so confused. And still in shock. What I managed to say was that I needed a home pregnancy test. Doctors made mistakes, right?

An hour later, I stared at the pregnancy test strip confirming that what my doctor said was true. I was going to have a baby.

After the shock abated, we shared our news with a few close friends, but only in strict confidence, not to spread the word. Mixed emotions gave way to excitement.

I was going to have a baby!

Since it was so close to Christmas, we decided to

wait until Christmas Day to share the good news with family. Because we lived 500 miles from my parents, that meant a special phone call Christmas morning.

"Mom, I have some news. Are you sitting down?"

"What's wrong, Amy?" my mom's voice quivered.

"Nothing. Everything is fine. It's just that I have a Christmas present for you that will have to wait for about nine months."

Silence.

Then Mom screamed and dropped the phone. I could hear her in the background, "I'm going to be a grandma! Amy's having a baby!"

My excitement grew.

Telling my husband's parents was a little more nerve-wracking. They had a better picture of our financial state, and I was afraid they would be more concerned about how we'd afford a baby than being excited for us.

Christmas evening passed in a blur. After the last present was opened, David spoke. "Mother and Dad, we have another present for you."

"But it'll be nine months before we can give it to you." I added.

Just as the last word left my mouth, my in-laws jumped off the couch and hugged us.

It finally settled in my heart. We were having a baby!

Then came the doctors' visits. Because of my diabetes I had to see a perinatologist. The only words that registered from that first meeting were, "You have a 40 percent chance of losing this baby if your blood sugar control isn't perfect."

Perfect?

I left in tears. Now I really didn't like doctors.

So I set out to prove that specialist wrong. I found a wonderful endocrinologist who helped me manage my diabetes well. Determined to beat that perinatologist's depressing odds, I worked hard to have a healthy baby.

Meanwhile, my first trimester nausea gave way to my second trimester nausea. Veteran moms promised it would pass soon. I tried Sea-Bands, ginger tea, and small snacks throughout the day. Nothing worked. And the doctors didn't help.

The midwives, on the other hand, were wonderful. They listened to my fears about all the things that didn't match up with the *What to Expect When You're Expecting* book I read daily. And they didn't balk when I stepped on the scale during my monthly visits. Unlike my perinatologist.

On one particularly fun visit, he said, "Mrs. Wallace, you really need to watch your weight." The shock must have registered on my face because he softened his tone. "It's just that you're young, and you'll want to get back to your pre-pregnancy figure quickly. So try to keep an eye on it."

Twenty-seven years of watching my weight left me wanting to use his head as a racquetball. I didn't. I behaved myself.

I was also still throwing up daily, and I was well into my third trimester.

The doctor just shrugged and smiled. "It'll end soon." I didn't see anything to smile about.

Then monthly visits turned into weekly ones, and my love for doctors diminished with every appointment. A girl can only take stepping on the scale with an audience so many times.

The ultrasounds were a saving grace. In the last few months, seeing my little girl growing inside of me gave me a new appreciation for my perinatologist. As I watched my baby suck her thumb and cover her little face, I knew every difficult doctor appointment had been worth it.

The visits were almost over. Soon I'd hold my little girl in my arms.

In the final few weeks, the praise for how healthy my baby looked lessened my disdain for doctors. They still weren't my favorite people, but they'd moved up my list a few spaces.

When weeks of walking every night and lounging in the pool till I looked like a prune failed to bring on labor, a necessary induction was scheduled. Due to my diabetes, my perinatologist wouldn't let me go past my delivery date. By then, I rivaled Shamu for size and welcomed the perinatologist's insistence on scheduling the arrival of my little girl. My doctor moved up a few more spaces on my list of favorite people.

When delivery day came, I checked my bags more than a dozen times before we left for the hospital. I made sure I'd packed gum, socks, my toothbrush, and my going-home outfit. Not my favorite blue jeans either. I also packed the adorable pink outfit my mom bought for our little one. And, per my husband's request, a nice white one in case the doctors were wrong.

As I waited for my little one to arrive, my husband and I played cards, watched TV, and with every contraction, watched all the monitors. Before long, the little line that monitored my contractions went way up and then down every few minutes. I was ready to be done.

No more cards, no more TV. Just a lot of breathing and hoping the clock would speed up to the minute my little one's scream would fill the room.

When my doctor came in and ordered my epidural, he shot to the top of my favorites list.

After the epidural took effect, I watched the monitors and laughed with every contraction. "I bet that one would have been a doozy."

A little while later a nurse checked my progress. "Are you ready to push?" She asked. Then she turned down my epidural. I wasn't too thrilled with that. "Doctor's orders. It'll help you take an active part in the delivery process."

My doctor slipped a few lines from his high place on my list. But when he came in to check on me, I was a little too preoccupied with pushing to let him know what I thought about my epidural being turned down.

Two long hours and little progress later, my peri-natologist said the words I dreaded most, "We need to do a C-section."

In a flash, my room filled with people prepping me for surgery. I cried hot, angry tears. This was not how I wanted my big day to go. But at least they turned my epidural back up.

The sterile operating room felt cold and lonely. My husband made sure the blankets covering my chest were comfortable and tried to soothe me with a play-by-play of all that was happening on the other side of the curtain. It didn't help.

I tried to figure out what I could have done differently during delivery. Or better yet, what my doctor should have done differently.

Then I heard it. My daughter's full-fledged, Richter-scale scream filled the room. I cried. She was here!

They placed her screaming form into my husband's arms, and he brought her to see me. He held her up to my face, and I cried as I spoke. "Elizabeth, Mommy and Daddy love you so much. We're so glad you're here." I looked at her round, little face and her head full of thick, dark hair. "You are beautiful, sweet girl."

Elizabeth's crying stopped. Her beautiful blue eyes focused on me. She knew my voice. With awe, I touched each little finger and stroked her silky cheek.

The doctor interrupted my revelry. "Congratulations, Mrs. Wallace. Enjoy your little girl."

I beamed.

Did I mention how much I like doctors?

Three times I would visit that operating room to deliver each of my precious daughters, the last two times with an obstetrician who made medical appointments feel like a day at the park. We'd joke about the latest movies, and he'd compliment my older girls on how well-behaved they were. With my last baby, I made it to the top of his list. At eleven pounds, eight ounces, my Sarah was the largest baby he'd ever delivered.

Despite their chart-topping size, all three of my girls were healthy, beautiful bundles of joy. I'm forever grateful for the doctors who helped me bring them safely into this world.

My middle daughter, Hannah, recently announced she wants to go to medical school when she grows up. "To help people," she said.

I smiled. Good thing I now think doctors are a mom's best friend.

—*Amy Wallace*

A Baby Shower Story

Birds serenaded as Mom and I ascended the front porch steps of my friend's suburban home. I breathed deeply, inhaling all of Earth's beauty. On the nest myself, I felt at one with Mother Nature.

My friend opened the front door and welcomed me to my baby shower. Pastel bows adorned the living room chairs and matching twisted streamers draped the ceiling. A cake with icing booties claimed center stage on the dining room table. Then hug, hug, kiss, kiss all around.

"Why, you're all aglow!" another friend said. Several other guests nodded their heads in agreement.

"I loved being pregnant," one rotund belle chimed, waddling toward us.

"Are you kidding? It was misery!" another joined in.

All the hens flocked around as if I were spreading feed on the carpet. Cackles, whispers, and traditional Southern gossip filled the room.

A few of my friends who had no children looked surprised when they saw me. I knew their wide eyes were due to my increased size. If a front view of my massive belly shocked them, I would spare them a rear view. My hips, which only a few months earlier could easily fit into a size three, had widened to what felt like the breadth of a freight train.

One of my coworkers, dressed in a tight mini-skirt and low-cut blouse, approached and made small talk. "So, how have you been feeling?" she asked, staring at the place where my waistline used to reside.

"She can't answer you," I said, pointing to my belly.

The coworker lifted her eyes from my belly to my face and smiled. "Oh, I meant you, of course."

"Well, I feel wonderful."

The baby kicked three times in rapid succession, and the coworker looked as though she were watching the scene in *Aliens* when a hideous creature bursts from a man's chest.

"Doesn't that hurt?" she asked with a look of horror.

"Only when a foot pops out." I smiled. "Just kidding. You'll love being pregnant when your time comes." I raised my shirt just enough for her to see my protruding, cracked, and scabbed belly button and wide, silvery stretch marks.

She paled and backed away slowly.

I left her to deal with the shock of what might well be her fate one day and headed for the living room, my stomach whining from hunger. A massive pyramid-like structure, made from diapers wound together, teetered on the hearth, and pink lotion bottles peeked over the rims of overstuffed gift baskets. The hostess ushered me to a wingchair to open gifts. This could take all day, I thought, rubbing my palms together in anticipation.

Gingham dresses, lacey socks, bottles, pacifiers, board books, and booties abounded. I received three Diaper Genies, and the older women were amazed at the new-fangled technology.

"You mean it sucks the stench right out of the air?" Aunt Methyl had eyes as large as saucers. "Why I never!"

"These young girls today don't know how good they have it, Methyl. Imagine, no cloth diapers." Aunt Gertie raised her eyebrows. "And now they have diaper wizards to boot."

The hostess stood and clapped to get everyone's attention. "You're going to love the baby games, ladies."

An intense dislike for baby shower games quickly closed the generation gap. Everyone sat back into their seats, shaking their heads. I heard tongue clucking and heavy sighing as the hostess passed out pencils and notepads.

We played guessing games about the soon-to-be-born baby's weight and length. Then the hostess presented a tray of twenty baby-related items. We stared at them in silence. A loud snore erupted from the sofa, and Aunt Methyl jabbed her elbow into Aunt Gertie's ribs.

"What?" Gertie rubbed her ribs and looked at Methyl. Then she noticed everyone staring. "I wasn't sleeping. . . . I was coughing." Covering her mouth, she faked a delicate cough.

The hostess covered her tray of baby items with a towel and told us to write down as many as we could remember. Since the older guests probably wouldn't remember half the stuff and the younger ones probably wouldn't have a clue what most of the things were, I thought I might have a chance at winning. I tried to envision the tray. My mind went blank. I forgot that pregnant women also suffer from memory loss. My mother remembered five of the twenty and won a magnetic refrigerator note pad. At the word "refrigerator," my stomach groaned.

Experienced mothers shared their wisdom and sipped sherbet punch, while the prematernal crowd chatted about manicures and Hollywood weddings. I sat near a window and tried to pay attention, but was lost in all the contradicting advice. One woman touted Dr. Phil as the authority on child rearing, while another sang the praises of Dr. Sears and another of Dr. Spock.

"Maybe I'll just buy a Dr. Seuss book," I said. The women looked at me as if I'd lost my mind. "I've always admired his philosophy—little Cindy Lou Who, transforming that wretched Grinch with all her warm sentiment and her big googly eyes." Green eggs and ham came to mind, and my mouth began to water.

After they'd purged all their advice, the hens dispersed and I began to rise. One friend of a friend with a silvery helmet of hair gave me a full, denture smile, and then narrowed her eyes and leaned in close. "At least you don't have to do the deed for a while. That's a blessing in itself."

I blushed. The deed? Did she mean what I thought she meant?

"Always hated that part of marriage, but luckily my Henry didn't have the drive I've heard some of them do." She peered over her glasses and gave me a you-know-what-I-mean nod.

Who was this woman, and why was she talking to me about sex? And bless her antique little heart, but why on earth was she talking like it was a bad thing? I smiled and said something about the curtains, trying to change the subject.

"That's the same trick I used to use, doll." She patted my knee. "Whenever Henry got all fired up,

I'd just change the subject. Usually worked. He could be a real horny toad sometimes, though."

I choked on my sherbet punch. My eyes shifted left and right, searching for an escape.

"In the later years, it was better," she continued, lost in her memories. "Men are like Fords; they've only got so many miles in 'em. He hung in there longer than some of my friends' husbands did, but once it got to where he was shootin' pool with a rope, he gave up for good."

I felt faint. "Look," I said, pointing out the window.

As the woman turned her head toward the window, mumbling something about the evils of Viagra, I jetted to the dining room. I spent the next ten minutes trying to erase from my mind the imagery her words had induced.

The faint rumbling in my tummy had grown to a vicious groan, demanding sustenance. The mega-burritos with extra sour cream that my hubby had run out at midnight to get for me had long since worn off. So had the three fish sandwiches I'd had for breakfast. I was famished. I ate five platefuls of finger foods. Only the Code of Southern Manners kept me from raiding the refrigerator.

Someone handed me a plate of cake and ice cream. After inhaling it, I snagged my mom's plate. "The baby needs dessert, too," I said, looking like a lioness over her kill. While I sat there licking my chops, everyone basked in the light of my maternal glow.

I yawned and leaned back in my chair. The woman next to me caught my yawn, and then the woman next to her tried to suppress it when it snuck up on her. She clenched her teeth, her eyes watered, and then finally she opened her mouth in a wide, unsightly manner. I watched as the yawn passed from one guest to another, like The Wave at a baseball game. When the hostess yawned, I knew it was time to go.

Suddenly my stomach gurgled like a greasy drain on Liquid-Plumr. A cold sweat dampened my brow, and the room began to toss, like a ship, from side to side. I knew the feeling well. Struggling to my feet, I looked at my mother. "Mom. Bathroom. Now."

She grabbed my arm and led me to the bathroom, where I relinquished to the ivory throne all the food I'd just put into my stomach. Standing tall, I straightened my shirt and reminded myself that I always felt better after the midday hurl. I flushed the commode and moved to the mirror, which was not kind. *Come on, glow,* I thought, *don't fail me now.*

Patting my face with cool water, I began to feel better. I opened the door and extended an empty palm to my mother. "Powder," I said.

She handed me the powder like a nurse assisting a surgeon.

A few pats gave me some color. I stuck my hand back into the hallway. "Lipstick." After the application, I looked almost human again.

"Perfume," I said. A few spritzes.

"Breath mint."

Mom placed an Altoids in my hand.

I popped it into my mouth, and then exhaled into my palm. The smell almost knocked me out. "Better make it two."

After smoothing my hair and giving my cheeks one last pat, I stepped out into the hall. "Waddya think?"

"The glow has returned," Mom said with a smile.

She lugged the gifts to the car while I said my goodbyes. Once we were outside, I stopped her for a moment. "Thanks."

A puzzled look surfaced on her face.

"You changed my diapers, let me live through my teens, and paid for my wedding. You've always come through when I'm at my worst. Have I told you lately that you're the best mom in the world?"

She gave me a big hug. "Well, it helps having a perfect daughter." Then she pulled back and looked me in the eye. "How about some crab legs with garlic butter and a slice of key lime pie?"

My stomach purred in approval.

—*Shauna Smith Duty*

Here's Lookinatcha!

I was busy with my day, thinking about a thousand things at once, when someone stopped me with The Look. Gone were the thoughts of shopping lists, spreadsheet enhancements, and possible nursery colors that had previously occupied my mind. I was reduced to the humble human attached to the pregnant belly. All because of that kind, sympathetic, well-meaning, but intrusive and knowing look.

I first received The Look about three months into my pregnancy, when it became physically apparent that I was not just gaining weight. Oh, how I loved the attention! The Look meant I was special and revered, soon to be a most respected member of society: a mother. I didn't stop to consider what the other person was thinking; I knew only that The Look made me forget the morning sickness long enough to glow.

Soon The Look was popping up everywhere, and my enthusiasm for it dimmed. There is only so much glowing a girl can handle. And when I was half-naked in a fitting room, mid-yoga pose, or waiting in line for the restroom, I certainly didn't want the attention. Encountering The Look so often and from so many people started to cramp my style.

Despite the constant interruptions, I tried my best to appease the strangers with regal humility. I adopted a geisha-style response so that I could escape quickly without too many questions or comments. I would dip my head, give a gracious smile, and clutch my rounding midsection with a slight furrow to my brow, hoping The Looker would assume that the baby was kicking the bejeebers out of my internal organs or that my churning stomach was about to let loose. (Sometimes, one or the other, if not both, was true.) And I'd make my getaway.

If I couldn't manage a quick escape, I would pivot my body in profile to try to avoid my ultimate fear in these situations: invasion of my personal space. Otherwise, as I quickly learned, some of The Lookers—after dispensing their probing questions, intimate comments, and unsolicited advice—would take it upon themselves to reach out and rub my belly. Ick!

Whether my belly got rubbed or not, these encounters inevitably ended with The Looker uttering some version of that tired, old line, "It goes so fast.

Enjoy it while they're little."

Easy for them to say! They weren't lugging around baby weight, aching hips, and swollen ankles. They already knew their children. I was more anxious waiting for my pregnancy to be over than a five-year-old is on Christmas Eve waiting for Santa to appear. I couldn't wait to meet my baby!

Baby longing was sometimes the motivation behind The Look, I'm sure. Little girls holding dolls gazed up at me with wide eyes, dreaming of their future. Busy younger women who had not yet begun the mother-hood trail looked at me and heard their clocks ticking. Mothers with older children were reminded that maybe there was time for one or two more.

Sometimes, The Look made me feel like I'd fast-forwarded straight into senior citizenship. Men stopped checking out my legs and suddenly began to open doors and carry my bags. My inner-feminist resented The Look, even though the help was nice.

Seeing The Look on my father's face was another shocker. *Oh no! Now, he knows for sure that I've had sex!* No doubt, he'd already figured as much; after all, I'd been married for three years. But one look at my bulging tummy provided glaring evidence of exactly what I'd been up to.

Most of the time, The Look came from women who were simply and sincerely trying to convey, with their kind words and that universal reserved-for-pregnant-woman facial expression, the indefinable wonder of becoming a mother. The Look came from women caught up in the throes of raising children and from older women whose adult children had long since flown the coop. My own grandmother stopped me cold with The Look after a Sunday dinner close to my due date. I had eaten too much and couldn't get comfortable. A nap sounded like heaven, and I almost didn't have it in me to sit and chat.

"It goes so fast," Granny said as she placed her wrinkled hand gently on my belly.

"I know," I said, nodding my head and placing my own hand on top of hers.

She turned her hand and clutched mine. The smile slipped from her face, and she pressed her lips together.

"It goes so fast," she repeated.

I looked into her eyes, and a chill raced down my spine. I looked at our hands joined together over my belly. One day, my hand would be the wrinkled one, and I would look out from eyes dimmed, but also wise, from time.

Suddenly, I got it. I knew what The Look meant. "I'll make the most of every moment," I said.

Now, a month after my daughter Maggie's arrival, I am trying my best—given my sleep-deprived, hormone-raging, frazzled state—to savor my time with her, knowing that these precious days and the years to come will pass quickly. And when I see an expectant mother in the mall or on the street, I can't help myself: I give her The Look and wish her well. It is my way of saying, "Welcome to the world of motherhood. It's the most amazing thing you'll ever experience. But it goes so fast. So hold on tight. Pay close attention. And enjoy every moment."

—*Jodi Gastaldo*

Sisters on a Sacred Journey

The still night is broken by the sound that wakes every mother from even her deepest sleep: a newborn's cry. I jump from my bed ready to take my newborn daughter into my arms only to find she is resting peacefully in her hospital bassinet. The little voice that woke me continues to call, and now there is movement behind the curtain that divides the hospital room. A crooning begins, soft and low, and soon the whimpering is replaced with the sounds of a nursing infant.

I stand looking at my sleeping daughter and love wells up within me. I watch the rise and fall of her chest in the dim light and listen to her breathing. Each breath draws prayers of thankfulness from my heart for this fragile life that has been entrusted to my care. I wonder whether the mother of the nursing infant sharing this hospital room feels the same way.

A new day dawns, and the other mother repeatedly flips through the television channels and then shuts it off. I cautiously pull back one corner of the curtain and ask if she would like to visit. We will be sharing this room for as long as it takes for our tiny, premature babies to receive the care they need and to become strong enough to leave. As I pull back the curtained wall separating us, I see that we two mothers, as well as our two daughters, are a study in contrast to each other.

My daughter's fuzzy hair is auburn, and her skin is white as a new moon. Her daughter's skin is the loveliest shade of brown, and her hair is shiny, long, straight, and black as the night.

"She's beautiful," I whisper, not wanting to wake our sleeping angels. "What is her name?"

"Mikaila Rain," she replies, her voice soft and filled with emotion. "What did you call her?" she asks, her long, thick braid falling over her shoulder as she gestures toward my baby.

"McKenna Mercedes … it means honorable and merciful."

My blue eyes meet her black eyes, and we smile. We begin talking, and I find she is eighteen years old to my forty-one. I'm old enough to be her mother, and yet we speak as sisters, for motherhood has made us ageless. We talk of the future, of our hopes and dreams for our little daughters, and find they are much the same.

She speaks of family traditions and powwows. In my minds eye, I see Mikaila with moccasin feet dancing to the rhythm of drums, wind blowing through her feather-adorned black hair, her hands raised to the sky. I imagine McKenna at recitals, *en pointe* in satin ballet slippers dancing to classical piano music, her hair pulled tightly back in a bun, graceful hands pale against the auditorium's darkness.

Both images fascinate me, and I want to ask the young mother more about her life, but a knock at the door brings visitors, and she is quickly surrounded by her familiars. The curtain is drawn and, that quickly, our connection is broken and we are again separate, as we are in the "real world."

But when her visitors leave, she pulls back the curtain again. I bring out some strawberries, a gift from one of my friends. We eat and talk, sharing news from the "outside," as though the hospital is a prison and we are inmates. I tell her about my husband waiting for me at home and the latest antics of my four other children. Her eyes take on a faraway look and she tells me there is no home, no family waiting to welcome her and Mikaila. She doesn't know where she'll go when she leaves the hospital. She talks of making a trip to Yakima, then possibly to Browning to see her mother, and then maybe on to Arlee in time for the next powwow. Abruptly, she decides it's time to shower and leaves our room. I've unknowingly

said the wrong thing and I don't know how to make
it right.

My thoughts are interrupted by Mikaila's cries.
*Should I pick her up and comfort her while her mother
is gone?* I take the gamble and lift her from her bassinet. I hold her close and rock gently back and forth.
She quiets down, and I rest my cheek against her
downy head. Born prematurely, she seems tiny and
incredibly fragile. I'm so wrapped up in the moment
I fail to notice the shower has stopped. I look up to
see her mother standing in the bathroom's doorway
watching me. I feel like a child caught with my hand
in the cookie jar and hope I've done the right thing.

"She was crying, and I thought I could help, since
McKenna is sleeping," I say, sounding as unsure as I
feel.

"Thanks." She smiles; and her eyes are happy.

This moment begins a trust between us that
grows with each passing day.

Time drags on agonizingly slow here, but as our
babies are growing and getting stronger, so is our
relationship. Finally, we are both given the news
that we are to be released the next day. I'm eager to
leave this place but find myself wanting to hold on
to this newborn friendship, which seems as fragile as
our daughters. We talk late into the night, knowing
the next morning will be filled with last-minute
instructions from the doctors and no time for us to

visit. She speaks of beading moccasins and making a headboard to carry Mikaila. It comes out that she has nothing for her baby—no clothes, no blankets, no bed . . . nothing. My heart hurts when I think of all I have collected in anticipation of my daughter's birth, and I want the same for Mikaila.

Long after we pull the curtain and retire to our own hard hospital beds, I lay awake and contemplate the situation. Mikaila is three pounds and almost three inches smaller than my McKenna. I realize that in a few short weeks I could pass clothes on to Mikaila. Its funny how intertwined our hearts have become as we've shared the highs and lows of life here. I want the same for our daughters, a friendship that could grow as they do, and the clothes would give us a way to stay connected. As we prepare to leave the hospital world, I cautiously offer the clothes and she happily accepts. We arrange to meet at the powwow in Arlee, and then, with one last goodbye, we part.

Our circumstances, our ages, even our looks couldn't be more different, and yet, our dreams, our hopes, our love for our daughters couldn't be more alike. I want to share with her clothes, blankets, memories, experiences—everything I am and anything I have. Sharing is what sisters do, and that is who we are . . . sisters, on this sacred journey called motherhood.

—*Phyllis Walker*

New Math

My knees felt weak, and I plopped into the nearest chair at the women's clinic.

"Are you okay?" The midwife, Laura, checked my pulse.

"Yes, I'm just a little surprised. I'm recently divorced and . . .

Laura nodded. "I understand." She smiled as she added, "You'll do just fine."

I wished I felt as confident as she did. My divorce had been finalized only recently. My daughter, Mena, had just turned two, and I was struggling to establish a home transcription business to support us. How would a pregnancy affect my new business? Could I earn enough for three people? Where would I find the time and energy to do it all?

My parents were horrified that I was pregnant out of wedlock, and withdrew all financial support and even rejected my phone calls.

My ex-husband pressured me to let him take Mena. He insisted I couldn't raise two children by myself. "She'll be better off with me, Ginger. Let me have her. It'll be easier for you with just one child."

As anxious as I was, I was equally determined to somehow find a way, and I refused to give up custody of my daughter. I began to feel resentment toward my ex-husband, and I was angry at myself for allowing an unplanned pregnancy. I was upset that I had to raise my children alone, and I felt more alone than I'd ever been in my life. I hadn't even had time to work through my feelings about the divorce. I wondered how I could ever love this baby as much as I loved Mena.

In that odd way perception has of calling attention to normal experiences and making them seem more vivid, it seemed like every woman in the world had a husband and children. I was haunted by happy traditional families. Everywhere I looked, beaming fathers tossed chubby little ones into the air as glowing mothers looked on joyfully. The child, of course, would be giggling with delight. I'd return home feeling lonelier and sadder than ever.

I was exhausted from working long hours to keep my business going, often in the middle of the night when Mena was asleep. Many nights I sat at the computer with tears rolling down my face as I transcribed. The worst part was the loneliness. While a new child was developing deep inside my belly, there was a hollow space within my heart. I worked alone at home with headphones on, transcribing court proceedings. I felt shut off from the world. Nagging doubts troubled me. How would I be able to care for this baby too? How could I even love it like I loved Mena?

As the baby grew larger, I withdrew even more. Trips to the grocery store and the clinic for examinations became my only contact with the outside world. I was so tired, and I wondered whether I had enough energy to even care for my daughter, much less another child. How would I do it?

Mena looked forward to becoming a big sister. I wanted her to participate in the baby's birth, so I checked out a video from the birth center's library to help prepare her, and a friend let us use her video player while she went shopping. The video was called Birthing in the Upright Position. The video showed a series of approximately a dozen South American women delivering babies. The "plot" was the same for each birth. The camera panned on a woman already in the squatting position, holding on to a rail. Within moments, the baby delivered into a pair of waiting hands. I spoke to Mena about the birth process throughout the video. I explained that it was natural and amazing. I made sure to emphasize that what we were watching was the final step in a long labor process.

When the video ended, I pressed the rewind button. Not familiar with VCRs, I didn't stop the video first, so we watched it as it reversed. One by one, the babies seemed to be sucked back into their mothers. Mena turned to me with a sincere expression and asked, "If we don't like the baby, can we put it back?"

Mena's fascination with discovering the world and her sweet spirit carried me through the long lonely months. Money became less of an issue, but I still wondered how I'd be able to love the baby. As weeks passed and my due date grew closer, my concern that I didn't have enough love became overwhelming. In tears one evening, I called Beverly, a dear friend and coworker at a previous job. She wasn't home, but her husband, Rick, answered the phone and he sensed my desperation.

"Hey, what's wrong? You sound like you're crying."

I poured my heart out.

"Rick, I don't see how I could ever love another child as much as I love Mena. How could I? I love Mena with every fiber of my being. There just isn't enough in my heart to go around."

"Ginger," he said softly, "When you have this baby, your love won't be divided; it will be multiplied."

His simple words calmed my fears. I knew he was right.

My parents came around before the baby was born, and we made an uneasy peace with each other. By the time I gave birth, I'd moved up in my job and become the primary transcriber for the court reporting company's owner. I earned enough money to cover my bills with enough left over to purchase the necessary baby supplies and a used crib. I decided to repaint it and chose a soft yellow base with primary colored nine-patch designs. While I was repainting the crib I realized that I had begun to love the baby.

I regained my sense of self-esteem. Each day, I felt more excited as I imagined what the new baby would look like. My new business associates sponsored a baby shower. I had everything I needed, except the baby. Mena and I were ready to see the new infant. Precipitate labor and delivery prevented Mena from attending the birth. The baby was almost born in the car on the way into town. I delivered my son, James, less than forty-five minutes after labor began.

James is eighteen now. When he was five, I met and married the love of my life, Phill. Since then, we've added two more children. Our home overflows with love for one another and for all four of our children and their friends. I smile now when I think back on the days when I feared I couldn't love two little ones. How right Rick was when he whispered those words that helped pull me through that difficult time: "Your love won't be divided; it will be multiplied."

—*Ginger Hamilton Caudill*

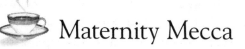

Maternity Mecca

Our New York apartment was so small we stored breakfast under our bed. Boxes of Frosted Mini-Wheats and Raisin Bran were crammed next to sweaters, winter coats, running shoes, roller blades, umbrellas, and other stuff that wouldn't fit into our one dollhouse-sized closet.

Because John and I didn't have the space for a bunch of baby things, I adopted a minimalist approach to maternity. While my friends had baby registries long enough to wallpaper their living rooms, I focused on just the bare essentials: a few clothes, receiving blankets, diapers, bottles. Even though my list was short, I was still looking forward to my pilgrimage to that maternity mecca—Baby World. Every expecting mother goes. Shopping at Baby World is part of the pregnancy right of passage, like feeling the baby kick or being offered a seat on the subway for the first time. Those who have been there claim that Baby World is more than just a store; it's a mother's best friend.

I celebrated the first day of my third trimester by driving to the part of town where the stores are as big as airports. With its giant, concrete, diaper-clad child holding a huge spinning globe, Baby World stood out among Home Depot, Office Max, and IKEA. I joined the congregation of pregnant women waddling across the parking lot toward the entrance. I had barely steered my row boat–sized cart through the automatic doors when, "Oh, my God, how cute!" I gasped. Baby clothes. Rows and rows of pastel blues, pinks, yellows, and greens— like a cotton candy farm. Little knit hats with fuzzy ducky details, adorable onesies with buttons like gum drops, and booties so yummy I wanted to pop them into my mouth. I put a few clothes in my cart. Then a few more. And a few more. As I uncontrollably grabbed clothes off the rack, I thought back to when I was shopping for my wedding dress. I had entered the bridal boutique with a firm budget in mind and left with a dress that could have been a down payment on a modest home—a home with human-sized closets.

Maybe I should put some clothes back, I thought. *But they're so adorable, and this is my first baby.* I decided to keep the clothes, but promised myself that I'd stick to the rest of my list. Content with my compromise, I went in search of bottles.

The store was as big as Costco and as magical as Disneyland. Huge stuffed teddy bears hung from the ceiling, the staff wore cheerful aprons, and street signs marked every aisle. I passed Lullaby Lane and Playtime Promenade and turned left down Burping Boulevard, which was full of bottle-related supplies. I examined a piece of equipment that looked like a Cuisinart; it was an electric steam sterilizer that, according to the box, "kills all household bacteria." I had planned to boil bottles in a pot on the stove. What if my baby dies because I killed only some household bacteria and not all household bacteria? I put a sterilizer in my cart. I picked up a bottle warmer and read the label: *Warm baby's meal with fewer trips to the kitchen.* I hadn't thought about how many trips to the kitchen I would have to make by warming a bottle in the microwave. If a bottle warmer would simplify what would surely be a frantic life, I needed one.

By the time I got to the end of the aisle I had a lot more items in my cart, but I also had a lot more confidence in my mothering abilities with a bottle sterilizer, bottle warmer, bottle drying rack and organizer, bottle cooler, bottle tote, and bottle brush. Now, I only needed some bottles.

I looked up and saw that the entire wall in the back of the store, from Diaper Drive to Learning

Lane, five Baby World blocks, was full of bottles. I took a deep breath and approached. I had no idea there were so many different kinds of bottles from so many different manufacturers. I became overwhelmed as I read the labels, searching for any intelligible information that would enable me to decide what to buy. Slow drip, fast drip, wide necks, infant grips, anti-vacuum valves, internal vents, training handles, vented nipples, anti-colic nipples, orthodontic nipples.

"Help!"

A sales clerk rushed over. She was wearing a yellow ducky printed apron with a yellow baseball cap that had a duck's beak substituting for the rim.

"I just need a bottle," I pleaded. "Which one is best?" Even though I was sure the sales clerk was a high school student working part-time and not an experienced mother, I was desperate enough to go with whatever she recommended.

"Well, it all depends on what your baby prefers," she said.

What my baby prefers? Had I heard correctly?

I thought for a minute, then asked, "Even if my baby does prefer the slow drip bottle with the vented nipple and anti-vacuum valve over the fast drip one with the orthodontic nipple and internal vents, how would I know?"

The sales clerk looked confused.

"He's a baby," I clarified. "He can't talk. But maybe you sell baby mind-reading machines?" I half expected the sales clerk to direct me to ESP Avenue, but she slinked away instead.

The wall-o-bottles was way too much frosting on the cake, prompting me to question what, if anything, was really underneath. I stared at the pile of stuff in my cart. So much stuff for one tiny baby. Stuff that, until coming to Baby World, I didn't know existed let alone that I needed them. A mother's best friend, I scoffed. An enterprise that preys on emotions and insecurities was more like it.

I walked out of Baby World, leaving behind my entire cart full of stuff, right in the middle of Splish Splash Street. I decided to do my baby shopping the old-fashioned way. I went to Walgreens. The baby section there was labeled "Baby Section" and took up only half of aisle three. I found everything I needed: blankets, diapers, and two bottles to choose from, a blue one and a pink one. Finally, a decision I could make with confidence. Three months later, Gregory was born. Just as I had hoped, he liked the blue bottle just fine.

—*Elizabeth Ridley*

"Maternity Mecca" was first published in the February 2005 issue of the e-zine *Defenestration*.

Welcome se,
Your Highness

I'll take the Bratt Decor spindle crib, antique white, please, with the matching chenille canopy. Oh, and that darling hand-pieced crib quilt. There must be a matching crib skirt too." I pointed out the items to the saleswoman.

"Have you considered the coordinating changing table and chaise longue?" she suggested.

Why not? I thought. *This has been a long time coming. My first real baby nursery. For my second baby. Why not?* I asked myself again.

Then something caught my eye. Tucked away in a far corner of that exclusive children's shop, lying haphazardly on a high shelf, was an infant car seat. This wasn't the deluxe model, leather, convertible infant carrier. No, it was the cheapest model available: a discontinued, grey, molded-plastic infant car seat with purple velour lining. At that moment, clear as day, I saw my baby in that car seat, my first baby, years before. . . .

The apartment my husband and I lived in years ago was modest. If I opened the closet door in the bedroom, there was no way to get to the dresser. If I opened a dresser drawer, there was no way to get to the bed. The toilet leaked, the carpet smelled like kitty litter, and occasional trains from a nearby railroad racked the shabby apartment.

Enter pregnant me.

"We'll make room for the baby," I assured my wary husband. "We'll move our dresser to the living room. The baby's crib will go in its place."

"What about the baby's clothes, diapers, toys, and other things?" My husband was skeptical.

"My desk," I offered. "I won't be working as much when the baby comes. I'll clear out my desk in the hall and put the baby's stuff in there. It'll work out fine."

Somehow, I would make our hovel a home.

I got to work. Some women get a sudden burst of energy a few weeks before delivery. "Nesting urge," they call it. I nested for my entire second and third trimesters. I learned to crochet. Since I only knew the basic stitch and couldn't quite catch on to the double joining stitch, I ended up with a pink wool chain long enough to wrap around Rhode Island. Twice. I alphabetized my spice rack. *Should lemon pepper go under L for Lemon or P for Pepper?* I puzzled. I embroidered a baby blanket, naming all the periodical elements and their atomic numbers (Zr, Zirconium; Co, Cobalt, etc.).

I also devoured every book on birth and baby care from our local library. The staff cringed when I entered each day: *Here comes the fat lady with the overdue list the size of the USS Constitution.*

At night in bed, I pondered the pros and cons of disposable versus cloth diapers. In the morning at breakfast, munching whole grain cereal and the recommended daily allowance of vitamins A, B, C, D, E, and the rest of the lot, I reviewed my notes from childbirth preparation class. I memorized my breathing patterns, anesthesia options, and breast-feeding latching techniques. The Lamaze books mention optical stimulation as a tool for cognitive development in newborns. So I painted black and white circles on our bedroom walls. When my husband complained that the walls kept him awake at night, I repainted them powder blue.

I had everything planned. Everything was ready. I needed just one final detail—the baby. We waited. And waited. (This is where the chain crochet thing really took off.)

A week after my due date, at my forty-one-week appointment, my midwife asked me, "Are you ready to have this baby?"

I lowered my eyes. "I kind of like the baby in here," I replied, rubbing my swollen belly. "I love this baby so much already. The little kicks in my ribs when I lie on my right side. The hiccups the baby gets in the middle of the night. The little pointed elbow that juts out just so. The baby is safe in here. I don't know if I'm ready to let this baby go."

"The baby is waiting for you, Cristy," my midwife said, laying a gentle hand on my shoulder. "When you decide you're ready, the baby will come."

After my appointment that evening, I looked around at our shabby little apartment—and had a meltdown. *It's so small! It's so ugly! A hand-me-down crib and mismatched sheets and blankets! A desk for a dresser! Our baby has no bedroom, no playroom, and no yard. What have I done? I tormented myself. This sweet, little innocent infant deserves a castle. A kingdom. Not a run-down apartment overlooking a parking lot.* I cried myself to sleep next to my baby's hand-me-down crib.

That night the baby came. My first, my sweetness, my daughter. Finally, I touched the little foot that kicked my ribs. Kissed the little mouth that hiccupped in the night. Stroked the little elbow that jutted out just so. My baby was here. While I was waiting for her, she had been waiting for me.

The next day, my husband and I drove our baby girl home. We pulled into the parking lot of our apartment. I unbuckled the baby's car seat from the seatbelt. She slept soundly, snuggled in that grey plastic car seat with the purple velour lining. I carried her car seat like it held a priceless crystal vase.

Then, something miraculous occurred. That apartment building, that homely box of bricks, transformed before my eyes. The old oak tree outside the main entrance—could I hang a baby swing there? And look how the bright sun pours into our kitchen window. The worn hall carpet seemed somehow comforting, the cracked plaster walls charming. Even our miniscule bedroom felt cozy, rather than crowded. How quaint our apartment seemed now, with a baby in it. How much more like a home. Our home.

In her car seat, her royal throne, our little princess opened her clear blue eyes and for the very first time looked directly into mine. And then I understood. My baby didn't want or need a perfectly coordinated nursery ensemble or a fancy mansion. All she really wanted and needed was my love.

—Cristy L. Trandahl

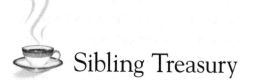 Sibling Treasury

"Mommy, when the baby comes, will you still love me?"

My five-year-old son's words stopped me in my motions of making dinner. I turned from the stove and looked down at Chris, standing there in his Superman Underoos and the little red cape I'd made for him, looking as anxious as a superhero who'd just lost his special powers. (Chris was always dressing up. One week he was Superman, then Spiderman, then a cowboy, then a pirate.) My heart melted.

It hadn't occurred to me before that Chris might feel threatened by the new baby, but suddenly I realized what my having another child meant to my firstborn. Chris would no longer be the sole recipient of his father's and my attention and love. In fact, he'd already been sharing us with his unborn sibling during the past several months as we prepared for our new arrival. To Chris, watching his toy room turned into a nursery filled with new furniture and wonderful new gadgets must have been like watching Christmas morning from outside the window.

Holding onto the counter top, I lowered myself to my knees and pulled my knobby-kneed superhero into my arms. I held him tightly for several long seconds before whispering into his ear, "Of course, honey. Mommy will always love you.

"I'll love you both," I continued. "But you—," I kissed his cheek, "You're special. You are my first baby."

Then, as I ruffled his blonde hair, I said, "Now, go play. Dinner will be ready in a few minutes."

He gave me a weak smile, which did little to reassure me that I'd convinced him of my undying love. Then he turned out of my grasp and raced out of the room, cape flying behind him.

Later that night while I lay in bed, I thought about all the changes that had occurred in Chris's life and what I could do to make the transition easier for him.

The next morning after dropping off Chris at school, I headed to the store for supplies. When I picked him up later that day, I said, "Chris, can you help me with a project?"

"Ah, I wanted to play with Brian."

"You can go play with Brian if you want. I thought maybe after dinner we could make a treasure chest."

His eyes rounded. "A treasure chest! For what?"

"Well, I was thinking about how cute you were as a baby. And about all the amazing and funny things you've done—like when you received the student of the month award from Mrs. Blakesly. I was so proud of you! And when you turned your plate of spaghetti over your head. What a mess!"

He laughed. "I did?"

"Yes. I have pictures," I said.

"Can I see them?"

"Sure, after you're done playing with Brian. And then we can make a treasure chest and fill it with all your special pictures and awards and mementos— things you want to keep for a very long time."

To my delight, Chris wanted to start right away. Forget Brian. Of course, before we could start on the project, he had to change into his pirate costume.

We painted the cardboard box a darker brown and brushed it with black to make it look authentic. Then I cut two strips from an old leather belt and attached them to the box and lid with gold paper binder clips.

I was so proud watching my little guy, tongue trapped between his teeth, paint his name on the side. He squeezed his whole first name, Christopher, on the box; never mind that the letters e and r were smaller than the rest and angled upward.

Over the next several days we searched photo albums, toy boxes, closets, and desk drawers, looking for the most special items to go into the treasure box. We didn't want to fill it, because, after all, we did have many years of treasured memories still ahead of us.

A week or so later I asked Chris to help me with another project. I needed little hands, I told him. He sparkled with excitement, but disappointment faded his smile as I steered him toward the nursery.

Curiosity grabbed him, though, when he saw the four metal cake pans filled with blue, green, red, and yellow paint. I asked if he would like to dip his hands into the paint and then place them on the walls everywhere I had marked it with a penciled X. His eyes lit up. It took all of thirty seconds for him to change out of his school clothes and into his play clothes. We had a ball, making a trail of little hands that went around the baby's room. And I took pictures.

Afterward, we sat on the rocker, Chris in my lap, and admired our work.

"You know," I said, "the baby is going to love you for making this room super fantastic."

"He will? How will he know?" (Chris had decided the baby was a boy.)

"We took pictures, remember."

"Oh, yeah." His blue eyes sparkled up at me.

Then we talked about all the things that he, the big brother, could teach the baby; how to throw a baseball, how to get dressed, how to brush his teeth, and even how to eat spaghetti without getting it in his hair. Then we talked about how he'd be part of Mom and Dad's team in making sure the baby was safe.

The next day after we picked up the developed photos, Chris asked, "Mom, could I put one of the pictures in my treasure chest?"

My plan had worked.

"Sure, honey. That way, when the baby is older, we can show him who made his room so great."

"Too bad the baby doesn't have a treasure chest," Chris said. "We could put a picture in it too. Then he would have his own."

"You're right! And you know what? We can make him one. I think I have another box and some paint left over."

His lips widened into a Cheshire grin.

That night Chris placed the picture, along with his love, into the baby's treasure chest.

A few weeks later, my very own superhero painted his baby brother's name on the box: Justin.

When Autumn and then Jordon were born, we created treasure chests for them too. Four boxes now sit on a shelf in my bedroom closet. Even though all my children have outgrown their Underoos, they still take out their boxes on occasion to enjoy the memories and the love we put inside them together.

—*Dianne Gerber*

Tell Your Story in the Next *Cup of Comfort*!

W e hope you have enjoyed *A Cup of Comfort for Mothers to Be* and that you will share it with all the special people in your life.

You won't want to miss our newest heartwarming volumes, *A Cup of Comfort for Parents of Children with Autism* and *A Cup of Comfort Devotional for Mothers*. Look for these new books in your favorite bookstores soon!

We're brewing up lots of other *Cup of Comfort* books, each filled to the brim with true stories that will touch your heart and soothe your soul. The inspiring tales included in these collections are written by everyday men and women, and we would love to include one of your stories in an upcoming edition of *A Cup of Comfort*.

Do you have a powerful story about an experience that dramatically changed or enhanced your life?

A compelling story that can stir our emotions, make us think, and bring us hope? An inspiring story that reveals lessons of humility within a vividly told tale? Tell us your story!

Each *Cup of Comfort* contributor will receive a monetary fee, author credit, and a complimentary copy of the book. Just e-mail your submission of 1,000 to 2,000 words (one story per e-mail; no attachments, please) to:

cupofcomfort@adamsmedia.com

Or, if e-mail is unavailable to you, send it to:

A Cup of Comfort
Adams Media
57 Littlefield Street
Avon, MA 02322

You can submit as many stories as you'd like, for whichever volumes you'd like. Make sure to include your name, address, and other contact information and indicate for which volume you'd like your story to be considered. We also welcome your suggestions or stories for new *Cup of Comfort* themes.

For more information, please visit our Web site: *www.cupofcomfort.com*.

We look forward to sharing many more soothing *Cups of Comfort* with you!

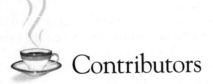

Contributors

Elizabeth Adam ("Moments and Miracles") is a writer living in Winnipeg, Canada, and currently working on a book about motherly love. She and her husband, Herb, enjoy Monopoly games and frog hunts with their two boys, who are almost six years apart and the best of friends.

Judy L. Adourian ("The Expecting Mother vs. the Accepting Sibling") lives in Coventry, Rhode Island. She teaches writing through her company, Writeyes, and is the executive editor of *NEWN* magazine and a member of the International Women's Writing Guild. Her work has been published in *A Cup of Comfort for Women in Love*, the *Providence Journal*, and *LitWit* magazine.

Mary Steele Allen ("Not Now") is a freelance writer and real estate agent from Greensboro, North Carolina. Her favorite pastimes are being a wife to husband, Steve, mother to three wonderful children, and Nana to grandson, Nolan. Mary's varied interests include church activities and painting children's murals.

Rose-Marie Barbeau ("The Wisdom Well") grew up in San Francisco with what her grandmother called an "itchy foot." After finishing an M.A. in international policy studies, she went on what was to be a sixteen-day visit to the Middle East that stretched into a ten-year stay. She now resides in Scotland.

Rebecca Bloomer ("All He Will Need") is an English/biology teacher from Australia. She has recently released a young adult novel about teen pregnancy called *Mae-be Roses*. Rebecca is also a Core of Life trainer, which enables her to deliver their pregnancy, birth, and early parenting courses to students all over Australia.

Anne O'Connor Bodine ("Boy Oh Boy!"), a former elementary school teacher, is currently a part-time freelance writer and a full-time mother. She lives in Evanston, Illinois, with her husband, Sam, and their two sons, Jack and William.

Amy Booth ("The Mother of All Jobs") graduated from University of California Santa Barbara and lives in Northern California with her husband and two children. She is a full-time mother by day and a childbirth, breastfeeding, and baby safety teacher by night. She is currently working on her first novel.

April Burk ("Waddling Down the Strip") is an award-winning writer whose work has previously appeared in eight anthologies and numerous magazines and newspapers. She lives with husband, Samuel P. Clark, in Archer, Florida, where their lives indeed changed forever when they hit the jackpot twice with daughters Kayla (twelve) and Sophie (six).

Jennifer Busick ("A Perfect Baby") lives in Owensboro, Kentucky, and writes for a living. Currently, she writes two monthly newsletters (the *Cal/OSHA Compliance Advisor* and *Day to Day Safety*), two monthly columns, and annual updates to her most recent book, *OSHA Training Guide for Medical Employers*.

Amanda Callendrier ("Baby Makes Four") currently resides in Buffalo, New York, and teaches writing at nearby Niagara County Community College. She holds an M.A. in English from Case Western Reserve University. Her husband and daughter keep her busy, and they are expecting a new addition to the family in 2006.

Wendy M. Campbell ("Not-So-Great Expectations") is a freelance writer and stay-at-home mother. As a former human resources specialist, she wrote business articles, and she now enjoys the lighter side of writing. She lives in the Pacific Northwest with her husband and daughters.

Candace Carrabus ("The Secret Club") is a writer who lives on a farm in the Midwest with her husband, daughter, two dogs, and seven cats. Her daughter, now six, delights and inspires her every day.

Ginger Hamilton Caudill ("New Math"), a native of Charleston, West Virginia, is a full-time writer who has been published in more than four dozen short story and poetry publications since October 2004. She writes a biweekly advice column called "Ask Aunt Henny," which is currently published in *Penwomanship* magazine and *www.cafeshe.com*.

Nancy Clements ("Mother's Intuition") is a mother of three living in Arizona. She works part-time as a self-employed contracted instructor but spends most of her time at her "real" job as a mom. She enjoys writing short stories and is currently working on her first novel.

Ellen Cullen ("Love Lost and Found") holds a master's degree in public administration, is a former government affairs professional, and currently works as a consultant. She lives in Northwestern Pennsylvania with her husband and son.

Amy Rose Davis ("The Flowers in My Garden") is a wife and mother of four children from Gresham, Oregon. To feed her creative writing habit, she enjoys working as a freelance copywriter for a variety of clients in the Portland-Metro area. This is her first published story.

Diana Díaz ("Just John") is a native New Yorker and single mother of two. She holds a B.F.A. in dramatic writing from New York University and an M.A. in English literature from Universidad de Puerto Rico. She works as the features editor for the *Caribbean Voice* and as an adjunct professor of English. Her articles have appeared in several publications, including the *Italian Tribune* and *Big Apple Parent*.

Peggy Duffy ("Picking up the Stitches") lives in Northern Virginia, outside Washington, D.C. She is the sales manager for a real estate firm and a freelance writer. She has published essays and short stories in regional and national magazines, newspapers, literary journals, anthologies, and online publications. Her monthly newspaper real estate column reaches more than 700,000 readers.

Shauna Smith Duty ("A Baby Shower Story") is a freelance writer and homeschooling mother of two in Roanoke, Texas. Though she loved being pregnant, parenting siblings that are fourteen months apart convinced her that a family of four was all the maternal fulfillment she could stand. She and her husband look forward to an empty nest and grandchildren they will spoil rotten.

Leslie Leyland Fields ("Too Many Ducklings?") is the author of five books, the most recent being *Surviving the Island of Grace* and *Surprise Child: Finding Hope in Unexpected Pregnancy* (*www.surprisechild.com*). She lives in Kodiak, Alaska, with her husband and six children, where she commercial fishes and teaches college English.

Jodi Gastaldo ("Here's Lookinatcha!") lives near Cleveland, Ohio, with her husband, Dan, daughter, Maggie, and son, Ben. She hopes to play the pregnancy game one more time but has to convince her cocaptain. He keeps mumbling something about preferring man-on-man coverage versus zone defense. Whatever that means.

Dianne Gerber ("Sibling Treasury") lives in Lehighton, Pennsylvania, with her husband, Jim. Between them, they've been blessed with five great children and two beautiful grandchildren (so far). An aspiring novelist with several manuscripts under consideration, Dianne also works as the corporate secretary for her family's fourth-generation trucking company.

R. L. Gibson ("Tea Parties Aren't Mandatory"), a married mother of one, is employed as a downtown development director for the town of Winnsboro, South Carolina. She also works as a freelance writer and special correspondent for the local newspaper. Her creative nonfiction and essays have been widely published.

Terri Reagin Gibson ("I'm Having What?) lives in Snellville, Georgia, with her husband, Phil, and those wacky triplets, Maggie, Robbie, and Pete. The only thing scarier than giving birth to triplets was sending them off to kindergarten, but now that the house is quiet for at least a few hours a day, Terri is writing a novel. This is her first published work.

Shanna Bartlett Groves ("Breaking the News to Grandma") is a Kansas-based freelance writer whose work has appeared in the *Kansas City Star*, *A Cup of Comfort for Sisters*, and *A Cup of Comfort for Nurses*. She has completed a memoir and is at work on another nonfiction book.

Tracey Henry ("Maternity Woes—er, Clothes") is a Tampa, Florida, area writer. She is editor-in-chief on *www.backwash.com* and writes the humor column "Suburban Diva." Her numerous published works include her book *Suburban Diva: From the Real Side of the Picket Fence*. She and husband, Sean, have three children.

Heather Lynn Ivester ("The Great Rabbit Chase") does more than chase rabbits; she's a columnist and author of *From a Daughter's Heart to Her Mom*. She's written for many newspapers and magazines, such as *HomeLife*, *International Living*, and *Christian Communicator*. She lives with her husband and brood of five children in Georgia.

Candy Killion ("Disassembling Momma Hen") is a freelance writer and the recipient of the 2005 Chistell Poetry Prize. Her writing has appeared in several publications, including *A Cup of Comfort for Women in Love* and *The Rocking Chair Reader: Family Gatherings* and *The Rocking Chair Reader: Memories from the Attic*. She lives in Davie, Florida, with her husband, John.

Mimi Greenwood Knight ("Why Didn't Anybody Tell Me?") is a freelance writer and artist-in-residence, living in South Louisiana with her husband, David, and four kids, Haley, Molly, Hewson, and Jonah. A frequent contributor to *Parents* magazine and *Christian Parenting Today*, she also has published her work in numerous magazines and anthologies, including *A Cup of Comfort Christian Devotional for Women*.

Gretchen Maurer ("High Fives All Around"), an educator and writer, lives in Ukiah, California, with her husband, Michael, and her three young children, Maya, Kai, and Noa. Her writing has been published in *The Discovery of Poetry*, *Adventure Cyclist*, and *Highlights*.

J. A. McDougall ("Our Journey Back") earned a bachelor of arts and a bachelor of commerce degrees from the University of Calgary. After working outside the home for several fulfilling years, she now raises her children full-time in Calgary, Canada. A few years ago, she began writing fiction and creative nonfiction.

Jean Mills ("A Friend in Deed") is the author of three children's novels, as well as numerous feature articles, personal essays, and book reviews. She teaches professional writing at Conestoga College and lives in Guelph, Ontario, Canada, with her husband and two children.

Cheryl Montelle ("The Procedure") started out as a dancer who sings in New York City and is now a mother who writes and teaches dance in Los Angeles. Her poems and essays have been published in *Fresh Yarn*, *Seven Seas Magazine* online, *On the Bus*, *Rattle*, and *Spillway*. She is the wife of renowned food photographer Brian Leatart and proud mother of Lily Rose Leatart.

Maria Monto ("An Old Wives' Tale") is the mother of three grown children, Lauren, Andrea, and Chris, and goddess to her two Bichon Frises, Buttons and Scooter. The former travel consultant resides in New Jersey and is currently working on a humorous short story collection. This is her second nonfiction piece to be published.

Juliet Johnson Opper ("Birth of a Nathan") has been published in *Los Angeles Family* magazine, the *Foothills Paper*, *MOMbo*, *Scribble*, and *Collages & Bricollages*. Her plays have been produced in five states, including off-Broadway in New York City. She lives happily with her husband, babies Nathan and Emma, and Gramma Moose in Los Angeles.

Janice Lane Palko ("The Master Plan") is a columnist, instructor, editor, and lecturer and a member of the Association of Personal Historians. Her many publishing credits include *A Cup of Comfort for Inspiration*. She resides with her family in Pittsburgh, Pennsylvania.

Gwyn Rhoades ("Basic Instincts") is a waitress, bartender, aspiring paramedic, and amateur writer living in Denver, Colorado, with her three children.

Elizabeth Ridley ("Like a Natural Woman," "Maternity Mecca," and "Tasmanian Tango") has been writing about motherhood since moving from New York City to Wisconsin to raise a family. She refuses to relinquish her expired New York driver's license, because she hasn't yet fully accepted her life as a Midwestern mom who buys diapers in bulk at Sam's Club. Elizabeth writes when she can and drives very carefully.

Estelle Salata ("All I Want for Christmas") is a Canadian freelance writer who frequently finds inspiration in her husband and children's experiences. Her stories and articles have appeared in 150 publications. The book she most enjoyed writing is *Mice at Centre Ice*, a middle grade hockey novel. Her latest book was published in three languages in 2004, by Stabenfeldt, Norway.

Laura Schroll ("A Daughter's Gifts") is a freelance writer whose essays and articles have appeared in national and regional publications, including *TEA: A Magazine*, *Byline*, and the *Detroit Free Press*. She lives on Long Island, New York, with her husband, Chris, and their daughter, Ella.

Piper Selden ("Waiting") lives in Hilo, on the Big Island of Hawaii, with her two children, husband, and geriatric cat. Her writing includes fiction, nonfiction, and poetry and has been published nationwide. Her work as an environmental educator makes Piper a popular public speaker, and she published a book on composting in 2006.

Emily Alexander Strong ("Charlotte's Web") taught middle school science before becoming a full-time mom of two daughters. An essay about her eldest appears in the anthology *It's a Girl*. Emily, her husband, Eric, and their daughters live in Ashland, Oregon.

Susan B. Townsend ("Baby Crazy") is a writer and stay-at-home mother. She makes her home on a 300-acre farm in southeastern Virginia with her husband, five children, and a zoo full of animals. Her nonfiction work has appeared in other volumes in the *Cup of Comfort* series, and her fiction can be found in numerous e-zines. She recently published her first book, *A Bouquet for Mom* (Adams Media, 2006).

Cristy L. Trandahl ("Welcome Home, Your Highness") has been a teacher and a writer for the nation's leading student progress monitoring company. Today she home-educates her six children at their home in rural Minnesota. In her spare time, she enjoys writing, fitness, and sorting socks.

Phyllis Walker ("Sisters on a Sacred Journey") resides in the beautiful Flathead Valley of northwest Montana with her husband and children, Britton, Matthew, Devin, Shae, McKenna, Shalom, and Tiana. She teaches piano, home-schools and writes whenever she can snatch a minute.

Amy Wallace ("Doctors Are a Mom's Best Friend") is a wife, mommy to three amazing little girls, and writer, living in Atlanta, Georgia. She writes to encourage moms in the most difficult, painful, and yet rewarding privilege of motherhood. Her work is also featured in *God Answers Mom's Prayers*.

Cynthia Washam ("Baby Talk") lives in South Florida with her husband and twelve-year-old son. When she's not listening to unsolicited advice, she writes for newspapers and magazines, including the *Los Angeles Times*, *Runner's World*, and *Surfer*.

Pauline Knaeble Williams ('When He Is New") grew up in a family of fourteen in Minneapolis, Minnesota. She now resides in Voorhees, New Jersey, with her husband and two young children. She is a yoga instructor and freelance writer.

Kimberly Charles Younkin ("Feeling Is Believing") lives in Columbus, Ohio, with her husband and their two young sons, ages four and one. She is a part-time, work-from-home freelance writer and ghostwriter whose tiny guys give her daily inspirations for writing and life.

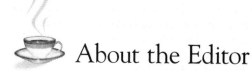

About the Editor

Colleen Sell is the editor of fifteen volumes in the *Cup of Comfort* anthology series. During her long career in words, she has been a book author, editor, and ghostwriter; magazine editor and features writer; journalist; tech writer; and copywriter.

The mother of three amazing children and three practically perfect grandchildren, she is anxiously awaiting the arrival of her fourth grandchild in 2006. She and her husband share a big old farmhouse on forty wild acres, which they are slowly turning into an organic lavender, blueberry, holly, and pumpkin farm in the magnificent Pacific Northwest.

The *Cup of Comfort* Series!

All titles are $9.95 unless otherwise noted.

A Cup of Comfort
1-58062-524-X

A Cup of Comfort Cookbook ($12.95)
1-58062-788-9

A Cup of Comfort Devotional ($12.95)
1-59337-090-3

A Cup of Comfort Devotional for Women ($12.95)
1-59337-409-7

A Cup of Comfort for Christians
1-59337-541-7

A Cup of Comfort for Christmas
1-58062-921-0

A Cup of Comfort for Friends
1-58062-622-X

A Cup of Comfort for Grandparents
1-59337-523-9

A Cup of Comfort for Inspiration
1-58062-914-8

A Cup of Comfort for Mothers and Daughters
1-58062-844-3

A Cup of Comfort for Mothers and Sons
1-59337-257-4

A Cup of Comfort for Mothers to Be
1-59337-574-3

A Cup of Comfort for Nurses
1-59337-542-5

A Cup of Comfort for Sisters
1-59337-097-0

A Cup of Comfort for Teachers
1-59337-008-3

A Cup of Comfort for Weddings
1-59337-519-0

A Cup of Comfort for Women
1-58062-748-X

A Cup of Comfort for Women in Love
1-59337-362-7